Welcome to ***"The ADHD & Autism Cookbook: 100+ Nutritious Recipes for Focus and Wellness."***

Why Nutrition Matters

Diet profoundly impacts the health and well-being of individuals with ADHD and autism. Proper nutrition can stabilize mood, increase concentration, and enhance overall physical health. This cookbook offers a pathway to improved focus and wellness through balanced, nutritious meals.

A Personal Journey

My journey began with my child, whose struggles with focus and sensory issues led me to explore dietary changes. The positive transformation inspired me to compile these recipes for others facing similar challenges.

What You'll Find in This Book

This cookbook features over 100 recipes designed to be nutritious and delicious. Each dish is easy to follow, rich in essential nutrients, and tailored to the dietary needs of those with ADHD and autism.

Key Features:

- Balanced Nutrition: Recipes packed with vitamins, minerals, and healthy fats.

- Simple Ingredients: Whole foods and accessible ingredients.

- Sensory-Friendly: Consideration for texture variations and mild flavors.

- Special Diets: Options for gluten-free, dairy-free, and other dietary restrictions.

Beyond the Kitchen

The book also covers mealtime routines, tips for healthy eating habits, and strategies for involving children in cooking. It aims to make mealtimes a source of connection and nourishment.

A Community of Support

You are not alone on this journey. This cookbook is part of a larger community supporting informed nutritional choices for the health and happiness of our loved ones.

Thank you for joining me in cooking our way to a healthier, more focused, and balanced life. Bon appétit!

1. Scrambled eggs with spinach

Ingredients:

- 4 eggs
- 1 cup fresh spinach, chopped
- 2 tablespoons milk or non-dairy alternative
- Salt and pepper to taste
- 1 tablespoon olive oil or butter

Instructions:

1. Crack the eggs into a bowl and add the milk. Whisk until well combined.

2. Heat the olive oil or butter in a skillet over medium heat.

3. Add the chopped spinach to the skillet and cook for 1-2 minutes until it starts to wilt.

4. Pour the egg mixture over the spinach in the skillet.

5. Let the eggs cook for a minute or two until the edges start to set.

6. Gently stir the eggs with a spatula, scraping the bottom of the skillet to scramble them.

7. Continue to cook and stir until the eggs are fully cooked but still moist.

8. Season with salt and pepper to taste.

9. Serve hot and enjoy your nutritious scrambled eggs with spinach!

This dish provides a good balance of protein from the eggs and vitamins from the spinach, making it a healthy option for individuals with ADHD and autism.

2. Oatmeal with berries and honey

Ingredients:

1/2 cup rolled oats
1 cup water or milk (dairy or non-dairy)
1/4 cup mixed berries (such as strawberries, blueberries, raspberries)
1 tablespoon honey (or to taste)
Optional toppings: sliced bananas, chopped nuts, or seeds

Instructions:

1. In a small saucepan, bring the water or milk to a boil over medium heat.

2. Stir in the rolled oats and reduce the heat to low.

3. Simmer the oats, stirring occasionally, for about 5 minutes or until they reach your desired consistency.

4. Once the oats are cooked, remove the saucepan from the heat.

5. Transfer the cooked oatmeal to a serving bowl.

6. Top the oatmeal with the mixed berries.

7. Drizzle the honey over the berries and oatmeal.

8. If desired, add any optional toppings like sliced bananas, chopped nuts, or seeds.

9. Stir everything together gently.

10. Serve warm and enjoy your delicious oatmeal with berries and honey!

This dish is packed with fiber, antioxidants, and natural sweetness from the berries and honey, making it a nutritious and satisfying breakfast option for individuals with ADHD and autism.

3. Smoothie bowl with banana, berries, and granola

Ingredients:

- 1 ripe banana
- 1/2 cup frozen mixed berries (such as strawberries, blueberries, raspberries)
- 1/2 cup Greek yogurt or non-dairy yogurt
- 1/4 cup milk or non-dairy alternative
- 1 tablespoon honey or maple syrup (optional)
- 1/4 cup granola
- Optional toppings: fresh fruit slices, chia seeds, nuts, shredded coconut

Instructions:

1. In a blender, combine the banana, frozen mixed berries, Greek yogurt, and milk.

2. Blend until smooth and thick. If the mixture is too thick, you can add a little more milk to reach your desired consistency.

3. Taste the smoothie and, if desired, add honey or maple syrup for extra sweetness. Blend again briefly to mix.

4. Pour the smoothie into a bowl.

5. Top the smoothie with granola.

6. Add any optional toppings like fresh fruit slices, chia seeds, nuts, or shredded coconut for extra flavor and texture.

7. Serve immediately and enjoy your nutritious smoothie bowl!

This smoothie bowl is rich in vitamins, antioxidants, and healthy fats, making it a great option for individuals with ADHD and autism. The combination of fruits, yogurt, and granola provides a balanced mix of nutrients to support overall health and well-being.

4. Greek yogurt with honey and nuts

Ingredients:

- 1 cup Greek yogurt (plain or vanilla)
- 1-2 tablespoons honey
- 1/4 cup mixed nuts (such as almonds, walnuts, cashews), roughly chopped
- Optional toppings: fresh fruit (such as berries or banana slices), chia seeds, granola

Instructions:

1. Scoop the Greek yogurt into a serving bowl.

2. Drizzle the honey over the yogurt.

3. Sprinkle the chopped nuts on top.

4. If desired, add any optional toppings like fresh fruit, chia seeds, or granola.

5. Stir gently to combine the ingredients, or leave it layered for a beautiful presentation.

6. Serve immediately and enjoy your delicious Greek yogurt with honey and nuts!

This dish is rich in protein, healthy fats, and natural sweetness, making it a great option for individuals with ADHD and autism. The combination of Greek yogurt, honey, and nuts provides a balanced mix of nutrients to support overall health and well-being.

5. Whole grain toast with avocado

Ingredients:

- 2 slices whole grain bread
- 1 ripe avocado
- Salt and pepper to taste
- Optional toppings: cherry tomatoes, radishes, red pepper flakes, olive oil, lemon juice, fresh herbs (such as cilantro or parsley)

Instructions:

1. Toast the slices of whole grain bread to your desired level of crispiness.

2. While the bread is toasting, cut the avocado in half, remove the pit, and scoop the flesh into a bowl.

3. Mash the avocado with a fork until it reaches your preferred consistency (smooth or slightly chunky).

4. Spread the mashed avocado evenly over the toasted bread slices.

5. Season with salt and pepper to taste.

6. If desired, add optional toppings such as sliced cherry tomatoes, thinly sliced radishes, a sprinkle of red pepper flakes, a drizzle of olive oil, a squeeze of lemon juice, or fresh herbs.

7. Serve immediately and enjoy your healthy avocado toast!

This dish is packed with healthy fats, fiber, and essential nutrients, making it an excellent choice for individuals with ADHD and autism. The whole grain bread provides sustained energy, while the avocado offers beneficial fats and vitamins to support overall health.

6. Cottage cheese with pineapple chunks

Ingredients:

- 1 cup cottage cheese (low-fat or full-fat, based on preference)
- 1/2 cup pineapple chunks (fresh or canned in juice, drained)
- Optional: a drizzle of honey or maple syrup, a sprinkle of chia seeds, or a few fresh mint leaves for garnish

Instructions:

1. Scoop the cottage cheese into a serving bowl.

2. Add the pineapple chunks on top of the cottage cheese.

3. If desired, drizzle honey or maple syrup over the top for added sweetness.

4. Sprinkle with chia seeds or garnish with fresh mint leaves if using.

5. Stir gently to combine or leave it layered for a lovely presentation.

6. Serve immediately and enjoy your tasty and nutritious cottage cheese with pineapple chunks!

This dish combines protein-rich cottage cheese with vitamin-packed pineapple, making it a great option for individuals with ADHD and autism. The combination of protein and natural sugars provides balanced energy, while the pineapple adds a refreshing and sweet flavor.

7. Egg and vegetable muffins

Ingredients:

- 6 large eggs
- 1/4 cup milk or non-dairy alternative
- 1 cup fresh spinach, chopped
- 1/2 cup bell pepper, diced
- 1/2 cup cherry tomatoes, halved
- 1/4 cup onion, finely chopped
- 1/2 cup shredded cheese (optional, such as cheddar or mozzarella)
- Salt and pepper to taste
- Olive oil or non-stick spray for greasing the muffin tin

Instructions:

1. Preheat your oven to 350°F (175°C).

2. Grease a 12-cup muffin tin with olive oil or non-stick spray.

3. In a large bowl, whisk together the eggs and milk until well combined.

4. Add the chopped spinach, bell pepper, cherry tomatoes, onion, and shredded cheese (if using) to the egg mixture. Mix well.

5. Season with salt and pepper to taste.

6. Pour the egg and vegetable mixture evenly into the greased muffin tin cups, filling each about 3/4 full.

7. Bake in the preheated oven for 18-20 minutes, or until the muffins are set and lightly golden on top.

8. Remove from the oven and let the muffins cool in the tin for a few minutes before transferring them to a wire rack to cool completely.

9. Serve warm or at room temperature. Store any leftovers in an airtight container in the refrigerator for up to 3 days.

These egg and vegetable muffins are rich in protein, vitamins, and minerals, making them an excellent option for individuals with ADHD and autism. They are easy to prepare ahead of time and can be a convenient grab-and-go breakfast or snack.

8. Overnight oats with chia seeds and almond milk

Ingredients:

1/2 cup rolled oats
1 tablespoon chia seeds
1 cup almond milk (or any milk of choice)
1 tablespoon honey or maple syrup (optional, for sweetness)
1/2 teaspoon vanilla extract (optional)
Toppings: fresh berries, sliced banana, nuts, seeds, or a dollop of yogurt

Instructions:

1. In a jar or bowl with a lid, combine the rolled oats, chia seeds, almond milk, honey (if using), and vanilla extract (if using).
2. Stir well to ensure all the ingredients are evenly mixed.
3. Cover the jar or bowl with a lid and refrigerate overnight, or for at least 4 hours, to allow the oats and chia seeds to soak and soften.
4. In the morning, give the oats a good stir. If the mixture is too thick, you can add a little more almond milk to reach your desired consistency.
5. Add your favorite toppings, such as fresh berries, sliced banana, nuts, seeds, or a dollop of yogurt.
6. Serve cold and enjoy your delicious and nutritious overnight oats!

Overnight oats with chia seeds and almond milk are a great option for individuals with ADHD and autism. This dish provides a balanced mix of complex carbohydrates, fiber, and healthy fats, which can help maintain steady energy levels and support overall health. The chia seeds add extra fiber and omega-3 fatty acids, making this a nutrient-dense and convenient breakfast.

9. Gluten-free pancakes with fresh fruit

Ingredients:
* 1 cup gluten-free all-purpose flour
* 2 tablespoons sugar
* 1 teaspoon baking powder
* 1/2 teaspoon baking soda
* 1/4 teaspoon salt
* 1 cup milk or non-dairy alternative
* 2 tablespoons melted butter or oil (or melted coconut oil for dairy-free)
* 1 large egg
* 1 teaspoon vanilla extract
* Fresh fruit for topping (such as sliced strawberries, blueberries, raspberries, or bananas)
* Maple syrup or honey for serving

Instructions:
* In a large bowl, whisk together the gluten-free all-purpose flour, sugar, baking powder, baking soda, and salt until well combined.

* In a separate bowl, whisk together the milk, melted butter or oil, egg, and vanilla extract until smooth.

* Pour the wet ingredients into the dry ingredients and whisk until just combined. Be careful not to overmix; a few lumps are okay.

* Let the batter rest for 5-10 minutes to allow the gluten-free flour to hydrate.

* Heat a non-stick skillet or griddle over medium heat. Lightly grease with oil or butter.

* Pour about 1/4 cup of batter onto the skillet for each pancake. Cook until bubbles form on the surface and the edges start to look set, about 2-3 minutes.

* Flip the pancakes and cook for another 1-2 minutes, or until golden brown and cooked through.

* Remove the pancakes from the skillet and repeat with the remaining batter. Serve the pancakes warm, topped with fresh fruit and a drizzle of maple syrup or honey.

These gluten-free pancakes with fresh fruit are not only delicious but also provide a good balance of carbohydrates, protein, and vitamins, making them a great option for individuals with ADHD and autism. The fresh fruit adds natural sweetness and extra nutrients, making breakfast a delightful and nutritious meal.

10. Quinoa porridge with cinnamon and apple

Ingredients:

- 1/2 cup quinoa, rinsed
- 1 cup water
- 1 cup milk or non-dairy alternative
- 1 apple, peeled, cored, and diced
- 1 tablespoon maple syrup or honey (optional)
- 1/2 teaspoon ground cinnamon
- Pinch of salt
- Optional toppings: sliced almonds, chopped walnuts, raisins, or additional diced apple

Instructions:

- In a saucepan, combine the rinsed quinoa, water, and a pinch of salt. Bring to a boil over medium-high heat.

- Reduce the heat to low, cover, and simmer for about 15 minutes, or until the quinoa is cooked and the water is absorbed.

- In another saucepan, combine the milk (or non-dairy alternative), diced apple, maple syrup or honey (if using), and ground cinnamon. Bring to a simmer over medium heat.

- Once the milk mixture is simmering, stir in the cooked quinoa.

- Cook for an additional 5-7 minutes, stirring occasionally, until the mixture thickens to your desired consistency.

- Taste and adjust sweetness if needed by adding more maple syrup or honey.

- Remove the quinoa porridge from the heat and let it cool slightly.

- Serve the quinoa porridge warm, topped with additional diced apple, sliced almonds, chopped walnuts, or raisins if desired.

This quinoa porridge with cinnamon and apple is packed with protein, fiber, and essential nutrients, making it an excellent option for individuals with ADHD and autism. The combination of quinoa, apple, and cinnamon provides a comforting and satisfying breakfast that can help maintain steady energy levels throughout the day.

11. Apple slices with almond butter

Ingredients:

- 1 apple (any variety you prefer)
- 2 tablespoons almond butter (or any nut or seed butter of your choice)
- Optional toppings: honey, cinnamon, shredded coconut, chopped nuts, raisins, or dark chocolate chips

Instructions:

- Wash the apple and pat it dry with a clean towel.

- Core the apple and cut it into thin slices or wedges.

- Spread each apple slice with a thin layer of almond butter. If desired, drizzle honey over the almond butter or sprinkle cinnamon on top for extra flavor.

- Add any optional toppings you like, such as shredded coconut, chopped nuts, raisins, or dark chocolate chips.

- Arrange the apple slices on a plate or serving dish.

- Serve immediately and enjoy your delicious and nutritious apple slices with almond butter!

This simple snack is rich in fiber, healthy fats, and essential nutrients, making it a great option for individuals with ADHD and autism. The combination of apple and almond butter provides a satisfying balance of sweetness and crunch, while the optional toppings add extra flavor and texture.

12. Carrot sticks with hummus

Ingredients:

2 medium carrots, peeled and cut into sticks
1/2 cup hummus (store-bought or homemade)

Instructions:

- Wash and peel the carrots, then cut them into sticks of uniform size.

- Arrange the carrot sticks on a serving plate or platter.

- Place the hummus in a small bowl in the center of the plate.

- Serve the carrot sticks with the hummus for dipping.

This snack is rich in fiber, vitamins, and minerals, making it a great option for individuals with ADHD and autism. The carrots provide a satisfying crunch and natural sweetness, while the hummus adds protein and flavor. It's also a convenient and portable snack that can be enjoyed at home or on the go.

13. Rice cakes with guacamole

Ingredients:

- Rice cakes (plain or flavored, based on preference)
- 1 ripe avocado
- 1 small tomato, diced
- 1/4 cup red onion, finely chopped
- 1 tablespoon lime juice
- Salt and pepper to taste
- Optional toppings: chopped cilantro, sliced jalapeños, or a sprinkle of chili powder

Instructions:

- In a small bowl, mash the ripe avocado with a fork until smooth.

- Stir in the diced tomato, chopped red onion, lime juice, salt, and pepper. Mix until well combined.

- Taste the guacamole and adjust seasoning if needed.

- Spread a generous layer of guacamole onto each rice cake.

- If desired, sprinkle chopped cilantro, sliced jalapeños, or a sprinkle of chili powder on top for extra flavor.

- Serve immediately and enjoy your delicious rice cakes with guacamole!

This snack is rich in healthy fats, fiber, and vitamins, making it a great option for individuals with ADHD and autism. The rice cakes provide a crunchy base, while the creamy guacamole adds flavor and nutrients. Plus, it's a quick and easy snack that can be enjoyed any time of day.

14. Celery sticks with cream cheese

Ingredients:

- Celery stalks, washed and trimmed
- Cream cheese (plain or flavored, based on preference)
- Optional toppings: chopped nuts, dried cranberries, sliced olives, or fresh herbs

Instructions:

- Wash the celery stalks thoroughly and trim off the ends.

- Spread a layer of cream cheese along the inside groove of each celery stalk.

- If desired, sprinkle optional toppings such as chopped nuts, dried cranberries, sliced olives, or fresh herbs over the cream cheese.

- Arrange the celery sticks on a serving plate or platter.

- Serve immediately and enjoy your delicious celery sticks with cream cheese!

This snack is rich in fiber, vitamins, and minerals, making it a great option for individuals with ADHD and autism. The creamy texture of the cream cheese pairs perfectly with the crunchy celery, and the optional toppings add extra flavor and texture. Plus, it's a simple and satisfying snack that can be enjoyed any time of day.

15. Cheese cubes and grapes

Ingredients:

- Cheese cubes (cheddar, mozzarella, or any other variety you prefer)
- Grapes (red, green, or a mix of both)

Instructions:

- Wash the grapes thoroughly and pat them dry with a clean towel.

- Cut the cheese into bite-sized cubes.

- Arrange the cheese cubes and grapes on a serving plate or platter.

- Serve immediately and enjoy your delicious cheese cubes and grapes!

This snack is rich in protein, calcium, and antioxidants, making it a great option for individuals with ADHD and autism. The combination of creamy cheese and sweet grapes provides a satisfying balance of flavors and textures. Plus, it's a convenient and portable snack that can be enjoyed at home or on the go.

16. Trail mix with nuts and dried fruit

Ingredients:

- 1 cup mixed nuts (such as almonds, walnuts, cashews, or peanuts)
- 1/2 cup dried fruit (such as raisins, cranberries, apricots, or banana chips)
- 1/4 cup seeds (such as pumpkin seeds or sunflower seeds)
- Optional: dark chocolate chips or chunks, coconut flakes, pretzels, or cereal flakes

Instructions:

- If using raw nuts, you can toast them in a dry skillet over medium heat for a few minutes until lightly browned and fragrant. Let them cool completely before proceeding.

- In a large bowl, combine the mixed nuts, dried fruit, and seeds.

- Add any optional ingredients like dark chocolate chips, coconut flakes, pretzels, or cereal flakes if desired.

- Toss everything together until evenly mixed.

- Transfer the trail mix to an airtight container or divide it into individual snack-sized portions for easy grab-and-go access.

- Enjoy your homemade trail mix as a nutritious and satisfying snack anytime!

This trail mix provides a good balance of protein, healthy fats, fiber, and carbohydrates, making it an ideal option for sustained energy and focus. Plus, it's customizable based on personal preferences and dietary needs, making it suitable for a wide range of individuals.

17. Kale chips

Ingredients:

- 1 bunch kale (any variety)
- 1-2 tablespoons olive oil
- Salt, to taste
- Optional seasonings: garlic powder, onion powder, paprika, nutritional yeast, or grated Parmesan cheese

Instructions:

- Preheat your oven to 300°F (150°C).

- Wash the kale leaves thoroughly and pat them dry with a clean towel or paper towel.

- Remove the tough stems from the kale leaves and tear the leaves into bite-sized pieces.
- In a large bowl, drizzle the kale leaves with olive oil and sprinkle with salt.

- Toss the kale leaves gently to coat them evenly with the oil and salt.

- Arrange the kale leaves in a single layer on a baking sheet lined with parchment paper or a silicone baking mat, making sure they're not overlapping.

- Optional: Sprinkle the kale leaves with your choice of seasonings, such as garlic powder, onion powder, paprika, nutritional yeast, or grated Parmesan cheese for extra flavor.

- Bake in the preheated oven for 10-15 minutes, or until the kale leaves are crispy and slightly golden around the edges. Keep an eye on them to prevent burning.

- Remove the kale chips from the oven and let them cool on the baking sheet for a few minutes before serving.

- Enjoy your homemade kale chips as a crunchy and nutritious snack!

Kale chips are rich in vitamins, minerals, and antioxidants, making them a healthy alternative to traditional potato chips. Plus, they're easy to customize with your favorite seasonings and are naturally gluten-free and low in carbohydrates, making them suitable for a variety of dietary preferences.

18. Homemade granola bars

Ingredients:
- 2 cups old-fashioned oats
- 1/2 cup nuts or seeds (such as almonds, walnuts, pecans, sunflower seeds, or pumpkin seeds), chopped
- 1/2 cup dried fruit (such as raisins, cranberries, chopped apricots, or chopped dates)
- 1/4 cup honey or maple syrup
- 1/4 cup nut butter (such as almond butter, peanut butter, or sunflower seed butter)
- 1 tablespoon coconut oil, melted
- 1 teaspoon vanilla extract
- 1/2 teaspoon ground cinnamon
- Pinch of salt

Optional add-ins:
- Dark chocolate chips or chunks, Shredded coconut
- Chia seeds,Wheat germ, Protein powder

Instructions:
- Preheat your oven to 350°F (175°C). Line an 8x8-inch baking pan with parchment paper, leaving some overhang on the sides for easy removal.

- In a large mixing bowl, combine the oats, chopped nuts or seeds, and dried fruit. Stir to mix evenly.

- In a small saucepan over low heat, combine the honey or maple syrup, nut butter, melted coconut oil, vanilla extract, ground cinnamon, and salt. Stir until the mixture is smooth and well combined.Pour the wet mixture over the dry ingredients in the mixing bowl. Stir until all the dry ingredients are evenly coated with the wet mixture.

- If using any optional add-ins like chocolate chips, coconut, chia seeds, wheat germ, or protein powder, fold them into the mixture at this point.Transfer the mixture to the prepared baking pan and press it down firmly and evenly using a spatula or the back of a spoon.

- Bake in the preheated oven for 20-25 minutes, or until the edges are golden brown. Remove the pan from the oven and let the granola bars cool completely in the pan on a wire rack.

- Once cooled, use the parchment paper overhang to lift the granola slab out of the pan. Place it on a cutting board and slice it into bars or squares using a sharp knife. Store the homemade granola bars in an airtight container at room temperature for up to one week, or in the refrigerator for longer freshness.

19. Smoothie popsicles

Ingredients:

- 2 cups frozen mixed berries (such as strawberries, blueberries, raspberries)
- 1 ripe banana
- 1 cup Greek yogurt or non-dairy yogurt
- 1/2 cup milk or non-dairy alternative
- 1-2 tablespoons honey or maple syrup (optional, for added sweetness)
- Optional add-ins: spinach or kale leaves, chia seeds, protein powder, or nut butter

Instructions:

- Place all the ingredients in a blender.

- Blend until smooth and creamy. If the mixture is too thick, you can add a little more milk to help blend it.

- Taste the smoothie mixture and adjust sweetness if needed by adding honey or maple syrup.

- If using any optional add-ins like spinach or kale leaves, chia seeds, protein powder, or nut butter, add them to the blender and blend until smooth.

- Pour the smoothie mixture into popsicle molds, leaving a little space at the top for expansion.

- Insert popsicle sticks into the molds.

- Place the popsicle molds in the freezer and freeze for at least 4-6 hours, or until the popsicles are completely frozen.

- Once frozen, remove the popsicles from the molds by running warm water over the outside of the molds for a few seconds.

- Serve the smoothie popsicles immediately and enjoy!

These smoothie popsicles are packed with vitamins, minerals, and antioxidants from the mixed berries and banana, as well as protein from the Greek yogurt. Plus, you can customize them with your favorite add-ins to suit your taste preferences and dietary needs. They make a delicious and nutritious treat that's perfect for cooling down on hot days or enjoying as a healthy snack any time!

20. Sliced cucumber with tzatziki

Ingredients:
- 1 large cucumber, washed and thinly sliced
- 1 cup Greek yogurt
- 1/2 cucumber, grated and excess liquid squeezed out
- 1-2 cloves garlic, minced
- 1 tablespoon lemon juice
- 1 tablespoon extra virgin olive oil
- 1 tablespoon fresh dill, chopped (or 1 teaspoon dried dill)
- Salt and pepper to taste
- Optional: a pinch of paprika or cayenne pepper for garnish

Instructions:

- In a medium bowl, combine the Greek yogurt, grated cucumber, minced garlic, lemon juice, olive oil, chopped dill, salt, and pepper. Mix well until all the ingredients are fully incorporated.

- Taste the tzatziki and adjust the seasoning if needed by adding more salt, pepper, or lemon juice.

- Cover the tzatziki and refrigerate for at least 30 minutes to allow the flavors to meld together.

- Wash and thinly slice the cucumber.

- Arrange the cucumber slices on a serving plate or platter.

- Serve the chilled tzatziki alongside the sliced cucumber for dipping.

- Optional: Garnish the tzatziki with a sprinkle of paprika or cayenne pepper for a touch of color and extra flavor.

- Enjoy your refreshing sliced cucumber with tzatziki!

This snack is rich in protein, calcium, and vitamins, making it a great option for individuals with ADHD and autism. The cool and crunchy cucumber pairs perfectly with the creamy and tangy tzatziki, creating a satisfying and nutritious snack that's easy to prepare and enjoy anytime!

21. Turkey and cheese roll-ups

Ingredients:

- Sliced turkey breast (nitrate-free if possible)
- Sliced cheese (such as cheddar, Swiss, or provolone)
- Optional: lettuce leaves, spinach leaves, or other leafy greens

Instructions:

- Lay a slice of turkey breast flat on a clean surface.

- Place a slice of cheese on top of the turkey slice.

- If desired, add a lettuce or spinach leaf on top of the cheese for extra freshness and crunch.

- Starting from one end, tightly roll up the turkey, cheese, and any optional greens into a cylinder shape.

- Secure the roll-up with a toothpick if needed to hold it together.

- Repeat the process with the remaining turkey slices, cheese slices, and optional greens.

- Arrange the turkey and cheese roll-ups on a serving plate or platter.

- Serve immediately and enjoy your delicious and protein-packed snack!

These turkey and cheese roll-ups are rich in protein and calcium, making them a nutritious and satisfying option for individuals with ADHD and autism. Plus, they're easy to customize with your favorite cheese and greens, and they can be made ahead of time for a convenient grab-and-go snack.

22. Quinoa salad with vegetables and feta

Ingredients:

- 1 cup quinoa, rinsed
- 2 cups water or vegetable broth
- 1 cup cherry tomatoes, halved
- 1 cucumber, diced
- 1 bell pepper, diced
- 1/4 red onion, thinly sliced
- 1/4 cup Kalamata olives, pitted and sliced
- 1/4 cup crumbled feta cheese
- 2 tablespoons chopped fresh parsley or basil

For the dressing:

- 1/4 cup extra virgin olive oil
- 2 tablespoons lemon juice
- 1 garlic clove, minced
- 1 teaspoon Dijon mustard
- Salt and pepper to taste

Instructions:

- In a medium saucepan, combine the quinoa and water or vegetable broth. Bring to a boil over medium-high heat.

- Reduce the heat to low, cover, and simmer for 15-20 minutes, or until the quinoa is tender and the liquid is absorbed.

- Remove the saucepan from the heat and let the quinoa cool slightly.

- In a large mixing bowl, combine the cooked quinoa, cherry tomatoes, cucumber, bell pepper, red onion, Kalamata olives, crumbled feta cheese, and chopped fresh parsley or basil.

- In a small bowl, whisk together the extra virgin olive oil, lemon juice, minced garlic, Dijon mustard, salt, and pepper to make the dressing.

- Pour the dressing over the quinoa salad and toss gently to coat all the ingredients evenly. Taste the salad and adjust seasoning if needed.

- Chill the quinoa salad in the refrigerator for at least 30 minutes to allow the flavors to meld together. Serve the quinoa salad chilled, garnished with additional fresh herbs if desired.

This quinoa salad with vegetables and feta is rich in fiber, protein, vitamins, and minerals, making it a nutritious and satisfying option for individuals with ADHD and autism. It's also versatile and can be customized with your favorite vegetables and herbs, and it's perfect for meal prep or picnics.

23. Chicken and avocado wrap

Ingredients:

- 1 large tortilla or wrap (whole wheat, spinach, or gluten-free)
- 1 cooked chicken breast, sliced or shredded
- 1/2 ripe avocado, sliced
- Handful of mixed greens or lettuce leaves
- Sliced tomato
- Sliced red onion (optional)
- Hummus or mayonnaise (optional)
- Salt and pepper to taste

Instructions:

- Lay the tortilla or wrap flat on a clean surface.

- Spread a layer of hummus or mayonnaise (if using) over the tortilla, leaving a small border around the edges.

- Arrange the sliced or shredded chicken breast, avocado slices, mixed greens or lettuce leaves, sliced tomato, and sliced red onion (if using) evenly over the tortilla.

- Season with salt and pepper to taste.

- Carefully fold the sides of the tortilla inward, then roll it up tightly from the bottom to form a wrap.

- If desired, you can wrap the bottom of the wrap in parchment paper or foil to hold it together.

- Slice the wrap in half diagonally if preferred.

- Serve immediately or wrap in foil for a portable meal.

This chicken and avocado wrap is rich in protein, healthy fats, and fiber, making it a nutritious and satisfying option for individuals with ADHD and autism. Plus, it's customizable with your favorite vegetables and condiments, and it's perfect for a quick and easy lunch or dinner.

24. Lentil soup

Ingredients:

- 1 cup dried lentils (green or brown), rinsed and drained
- 1 onion, diced
- 2 carrots, diced
- 2 celery stalks, diced
- 3 cloves garlic, minced
- 1 can (14.5 oz) diced tomatoes
- 4 cups vegetable broth or chicken broth
- 1 teaspoon dried thyme
- 1 teaspoon dried oregano
- 1 bay leaf
- Salt and pepper to taste
- Olive oil for cooking
- Fresh parsley for garnish (optional)
- Lemon wedges for serving (optional)

Instructions:

- Heat a large pot over medium heat and add a drizzle of olive oil.

- Add the diced onion, carrots, and celery to the pot. Cook, stirring occasionally, until the vegetables are softened, about 5-7 minutes.

- Add the minced garlic to the pot and cook for an additional 1-2 minutes, until fragrant.

- Stir in the dried lentils, diced tomatoes (with their juices), vegetable or chicken broth, dried thyme, dried oregano, and bay leaf.

- Bring the soup to a simmer, then reduce the heat to low and cover the pot with a lid. Let the soup simmer for 20-25 minutes, or until the lentils are tender.

- Taste the soup and season with salt and pepper to taste.

- If the soup is too thick, you can add more broth or water to reach your desired consistency.

- Remove the bay leaf from the soup before serving.

- Ladle the lentil soup into bowls and garnish with fresh parsley, if desired.

- Serve the soup hot with lemon wedges on the side for squeezing over the soup, if desired.

This lentil soup is rich in protein, fiber, vitamins, and minerals, making it a nutritious and filling option for individuals with ADHD and autism. It's also hearty, comforting, and easy to make in large batches for meal prep or freezing for later.

25. Grilled cheese sandwich on whole grain bread

Ingredients:

- 2 slices whole grain bread
- 2 slices cheese (cheddar, American, Swiss, or your favorite cheese)
- Butter or margarine, softened

Instructions:

- Heat a skillet or griddle over medium heat.

- Spread one side of each slice of whole grain bread with butter or margarine.

- Place one slice of bread, buttered side down, on the skillet or griddle.

- Layer the cheese slices on top of the bread slice.

- Place the second slice of bread, buttered side up, on top of the cheese.

- Cook the sandwich for 3-4 minutes on each side, or until the bread is golden brown and crispy, and the cheese is melted.

- Press down gently on the sandwich with a spatula while cooking to help the cheese melt evenly.

- Once both sides are golden brown and the cheese is melted, remove the sandwich from the skillet or griddle.

- Let the sandwich cool for a minute or two before slicing it in half diagonally, if desired.

- Serve the grilled cheese sandwich hot and enjoy!

This grilled cheese sandwich on whole grain bread is rich in fiber, protein, and calcium, making it a nutritious and satisfying option for individuals with ADHD and autism. Plus, it's quick and easy to make, and you can customize it with your favorite cheese and bread for variety.

26. Spinach and mushroom frittata

Ingredients:
- 6 large eggs
- 1/4 cup milk or non-dairy alternative
- 1 tablespoon olive oil
- 1 cup mushrooms, sliced
- 2 cups fresh spinach leaves
- 1/2 onion, diced
- 1 clove garlic, minced
- 1/2 cup shredded cheese (such as cheddar, mozzarella, or Swiss)
- Salt and pepper to taste
- Optional: fresh herbs (such as parsley or thyme), for garnish

Instructions:
- Preheat your oven to 350°F (175°C).

- In a large mixing bowl, whisk together the eggs and milk until well combined. Season with salt and pepper to taste. Set aside. Heat the olive oil in a large oven-safe skillet over medium heat.

- Add the diced onion to the skillet and sauté for 2-3 minutes, until softened. Add the sliced mushrooms to the skillet and cook for another 3-4 minutes, until they begin to brown.

- Add the minced garlic to the skillet and cook for 1 minute, until fragrant. Add the fresh spinach leaves to the skillet and cook, stirring occasionally, until wilted. Spread the vegetables evenly across the bottom of the skillet.

- Pour the egg mixture over the vegetables in the skillet. Use a spatula to gently stir the mixture, ensuring the vegetables are evenly distributed. Sprinkle the shredded cheese over the top of the frittata.

- Transfer the skillet to the preheated oven and bake for 12-15 minutes, or until the frittata is set and the cheese is melted and bubbly.

- Remove the skillet from the oven and let the frittata cool for a few minutes before slicing. Garnish with fresh herbs, if desired, before serving.

This spinach and mushroom frittata is rich in protein, vitamins, and minerals, making it a nutritious and delicious option for individuals with ADHD and autism. It's versatile, easy to make, and perfect for breakfast, brunch, or any meal of the day. Plus, you can customize it with your favorite vegetables and cheese for variety.

27. Chicken salad with mixed greens

Ingredients:
- 2 cups cooked chicken breast, shredded or diced
- 4 cups mixed salad greens (such as spinach, arugula, romaine, or kale)
- 1/2 cup cherry tomatoes, halved
- 1/4 cup cucumber, sliced
- 1/4 cup red onion, thinly sliced
- 1/4 cup bell pepper, diced
- 1/4 cup shredded carrots
- 1/4 cup crumbled feta cheese or goat cheese (optional)
- 2 tablespoons chopped fresh herbs (such as parsley, basil, or cilantro)
- Salt and pepper to taste
- Salad dressing of your choice (such as balsamic vinaigrette, ranch, or honey mustard)

Instructions:

- In a large mixing bowl, combine the cooked chicken breast, mixed salad greens, cherry tomatoes, cucumber, red onion, bell pepper, shredded carrots, crumbled feta cheese or goat cheese (if using), and chopped fresh herbs.

- Season the salad with salt and pepper to taste.

- Drizzle the salad dressing over the salad, starting with a small amount, and toss gently to coat all the ingredients evenly. Add more dressing as needed to reach your desired level of flavor and moisture.

- Taste the salad and adjust seasoning or dressing if needed.

- Divide the chicken salad among individual serving plates or bowls.

- Serve immediately and enjoy your delicious and nutritious chicken salad with mixed greens!

This chicken salad with mixed greens is rich in protein, fiber, vitamins, and minerals, making it a nutritious and satisfying option for individuals with ADHD and autism. It's versatile, easy to make, and perfect for a light and refreshing meal any time of day. Plus, you can customize it with your favorite vegetables, cheese, and dressing for variety.

28. Tuna and bean salad

Ingredients:

- 1 can (15 oz) white beans (such as cannellini or navy beans), drained and rinsed
- 1 can (5 oz) tuna, drained
- 1/4 cup red onion, finely chopped
- 1/4 cup bell pepper, diced
- 1/4 cup cucumber, diced
- 1/4 cup cherry tomatoes, halved
- 2 tablespoons chopped fresh parsley or cilantro
- 2 tablespoons extra virgin olive oil
- 1 tablespoon lemon juice
- 1 clove garlic, minced
- Salt and pepper to taste
- Optional: crumbled feta cheese, sliced olives, or capers for extra flavor

Instructions:

- In a large mixing bowl, combine the white beans, drained tuna, chopped red onion, diced bell pepper, diced cucumber, halved cherry tomatoes, and chopped fresh parsley or cilantro.

- In a small bowl, whisk together the extra virgin olive oil, lemon juice, minced garlic, salt, and pepper to make the dressing.

- Pour the dressing over the tuna and bean mixture in the large mixing bowl.

- Toss gently to coat all the ingredients evenly with the dressing.

- Taste the salad and adjust seasoning if needed.

- If desired, sprinkle crumbled feta cheese, sliced olives, or capers over the salad for extra flavor.

- Serve the tuna and bean salad immediately, or refrigerate it for at least 30 minutes to allow the flavors to meld together before serving.

This tuna and bean salad is rich in protein, fiber, vitamins, and minerals, making it a nutritious and satisfying option for individuals with ADHD and autism. It's quick and easy to make, and perfect for a light and refreshing meal any time of day. Plus, you can customize it with your favorite vegetables and toppings for variety.

29. Rice and black bean bowl

Ingredients:

- 1 cup cooked rice (brown rice, white rice, or quinoa)
- 1 can (15 oz) black beans, drained and rinsed
- 1/2 cup corn kernels (fresh, frozen, or canned)
- 1/4 cup diced red bell pepper
- 1/4 cup diced tomato
- 1/4 cup diced red onion
- 1/4 cup chopped fresh cilantro
- 1 avocado, sliced
- Juice of 1 lime
- Salt and pepper to taste
- Optional toppings: shredded cheese, salsa, sour cream, diced jalapeños, or hot sauce

Instructions:

- In a large mixing bowl, combine the cooked rice, black beans, corn kernels, diced red bell pepper, diced tomato, diced red onion, and chopped fresh cilantro.

- Squeeze the lime juice over the rice and bean mixture.

- Season with salt and pepper to taste, and toss gently to combine all the ingredients evenly.

- Divide the rice and black bean mixture among serving bowls.

- Top each bowl with sliced avocado.

- If desired, garnish with additional chopped cilantro and any optional toppings of your choice, such as shredded cheese, salsa, sour cream, diced jalapeños, or hot sauce.

- Serve the rice and black bean bowls immediately and enjoy!

This rice and black bean bowl is rich in fiber, protein, vitamins, and minerals, making it a nutritious and satisfying option for individuals with ADHD and autism. It's versatile, easy to make, and perfect for a quick and healthy meal any time of day. Plus, you can customize it with your favorite toppings and add-ins for variety.

30. Vegetable stir-fry with tofu

Ingredients:
- 1 block (14 oz) extra firm tofu, drained and pressed
- 2 tablespoons soy sauce or tamari
- 1 tablespoon sesame oil
- 1 tablespoon cornstarch
- 2 tablespoons vegetable oil, divided
- 2 cloves garlic, minced
- 1 tablespoon ginger, minced
- 1 bell pepper, sliced
- 1 carrot, julienned
- 1 cup broccoli florets
- 1 cup snap peas or snow peas
- 1 cup sliced mushrooms
- 2 green onions, sliced
- Cooked rice or noodles, for serving

For the sauce:
- 1/4 cup soy sauce or tamari
- 2 tablespoons rice vinegar
- 1 tablespoon sesame oil
- 1 tablespoon honey or maple syrup
- 1 teaspoon cornstarch
- 1/4 cup water

Instructions:
- Cut the pressed tofu into cubes and place them in a bowl. In a separate small bowl, whisk together 2 tablespoons of soy sauce or tamari, 1 tablespoon of sesame oil, and 1 tablespoon of cornstarch. Pour this mixture over the tofu cubes and gently toss to coat. Let the tofu marinate for at least 15 minutes.

- In a small bowl, whisk together all the ingredients for the sauce: 1/4 cup soy sauce or tamari, 2 tablespoons rice vinegar, 1 tablespoon sesame oil, 1 tablespoon honey or maple syrup, 1 teaspoon cornstarch, and 1/4 cup water. Set aside.

- Heat 1 tablespoon of vegetable oil in a large skillet or wok over medium-high heat. Add the marinated tofu cubes to the skillet in a single layer, making sure they're not overcrowded. Cook for 3-4 minutes on each side, or until golden and crispy. Remove the tofu from the skillet and set aside.

- In the same skillet, heat the remaining tablespoon of vegetable oil. Add the minced garlic and ginger, and cook for 1 minute until fragrant.

- Add the sliced bell pepper, julienned carrot, broccoli florets, snap peas or snow peas, and sliced mushrooms to the skillet. Stir-fry for 4-5 minutes, or until the vegetables are crisp-tender.

- Return the cooked tofu to the skillet with the vegetables. Pour the prepared sauce over the tofu and vegetables, and toss everything together until well coated. Cook for an additional 1-2 minutes, or until the sauce has thickened slightly.

- Remove the skillet from the heat and sprinkle sliced green onions on top. Serve the vegetable stir-fry with tofu hot over cooked rice or noodles.

31. Baked salmon with sweet potato

Ingredients:

- 2 salmon fillets (about 6 oz each)
- 2 medium sweet potatoes
- 2 tablespoons olive oil, divided
- 1 teaspoon paprika
- 1 teaspoon garlic powder
- 1 teaspoon dried thyme
- Salt and pepper to taste
- Fresh lemon wedges for serving
- Chopped fresh parsley for garnish (optional)

Instructions:

- Preheat your oven to 400°F (200°C).

- Peel the sweet potatoes and cut them into cubes.

- Place the sweet potato cubes on a baking sheet lined with parchment paper. Drizzle with 1 tablespoon of olive oil and season with paprika, garlic powder, dried thyme, salt, and pepper. Toss to coat the sweet potatoes evenly.

- Bake the sweet potatoes in the preheated oven for 20-25 minutes, or until tender and lightly browned, stirring halfway through.

- While the sweet potatoes are baking, prepare the salmon. Place the salmon fillets on another baking sheet lined with parchment paper. Drizzle with the remaining tablespoon of olive oil and season with salt and pepper.

- When the sweet potatoes have about 10-15 minutes left to bake, place the salmon in the oven and bake alongside the sweet potatoes for 10-12 minutes, or until the salmon is cooked through and flakes easily with a fork.

- Once the sweet potatoes and salmon are cooked, remove them from the oven. Serve the baked salmon with sweet potatoes hot, garnished with fresh lemon wedges and chopped parsley if desired.

This baked salmon with sweet potato is rich in omega-3 fatty acids, vitamins, and minerals, making it a nutritious and satisfying option for individuals with ADHD and autism. It's easy to make, flavorful, and perfect for a healthy dinner any night of the week. Plus, you can customize it with your favorite herbs and spices for extra flavor.

32. Chicken and vegetable skewers

Ingredients:
- 2 boneless, skinless chicken breasts, cut into bite-sized pieces
- 2 bell peppers (any color), cut into chunks
- 1 red onion, cut into chunks
- 1 zucchini, sliced into rounds
- 8-10 cherry tomatoes
- Wooden or metal skewers
- Olive oil
- Salt and pepper to taste
- Optional marinade: lemon juice, garlic, herbs (such as rosemary or thyme), soy sauce, or your favorite marinade

Instructions:
- If using wooden skewers, soak them in water for at least 30 minutes to prevent them from burning on the grill. Preheat your grill to medium-high heat or preheat your oven broiler.

- Thread the chicken pieces and chopped vegetables onto the skewers, alternating between chicken and vegetables. Brush the skewers with olive oil and season with salt and pepper.

- If using a marinade, you can marinate the chicken and vegetables in the marinade for 30 minutes to overnight before threading them onto the skewers.

- Grill the skewers over medium-high heat for 10-12 minutes, turning occasionally, until the chicken is cooked through and the vegetables are tender and lightly charred.

- If using the oven broiler, place the skewers on a broiler pan or baking sheet lined with aluminum foil. Broil for 10-12 minutes, turning occasionally, until the chicken is cooked through and the vegetables are tender and lightly charred.

- Remove the skewers from the grill or oven and let them cool for a few minutes before serving. Serve the chicken and vegetable skewers hot, with your favorite dipping sauce or alongside rice, quinoa, or salad.

These chicken and vegetable skewers are a nutritious and delicious option for individuals with ADHD and autism. They're packed with protein, vitamins, and minerals from the chicken and vegetables, and they're easy to customize with your favorite marinade and vegetables. Plus, they're fun to eat and perfect for a family-friendly meal or outdoor barbecue.

33. Beef and broccoli stir-fry

Ingredients:

- 1 lb flank steak or sirloin steak, thinly sliced against the grain
- 3 cups broccoli florets
- 2 tablespoons vegetable oil, divided
- 3 cloves garlic, minced
- 1 tablespoon fresh ginger, minced
- 1/4 cup soy sauce or tamari
- 2 tablespoons oyster sauce
- 1 tablespoon hoisin sauce
- 1 tablespoon cornstarch
- 1/4 cup water or beef broth
- Cooked rice or noodles, for serving
- Sesame seeds and sliced green onions for garnish (optional)

Instructions:

- In a small bowl, whisk together the soy sauce or tamari, oyster sauce, hoisin sauce, cornstarch, and water or beef broth to make the sauce. Set aside.

- Heat 1 tablespoon of vegetable oil in a large skillet or wok over medium-high heat. Add the thinly sliced beef in a single layer and cook for 1-2 minutes without stirring to sear one side. Then, stir-fry for another 1-2 minutes until browned and cooked through. Remove the beef from the skillet and set aside.

- In the same skillet, heat the remaining tablespoon of vegetable oil. Add the minced garlic and ginger, and cook for 1 minute until fragrant.

- Add the broccoli florets to the skillet and stir-fry for 3-4 minutes, or until crisp-tender. Return the cooked beef to the skillet with the broccoli. Give the sauce a quick stir and then pour it over the beef and broccoli in the skillet.

- Stir-fry everything together for another 1-2 minutes until the sauce thickens and coats the beef and broccoli evenly.

- Remove the skillet from the heat. Serve the beef and broccoli stir-fry hot over cooked rice or noodles. Garnish with sesame seeds and sliced green onions, if desired.

This beef and broccoli stir-fry is a nutritious and flavorful option for individuals with ADHD and autism. It's rich in protein, vitamins, and minerals, and it's quick and easy to make. Plus, you can customize it with your favorite vegetables and serve it with rice or noodles for a complete and satisfying meal.

34. Quinoa-stuffed bell peppers

Ingredients:
- 4 large bell peppers (any color), halved and seeds removed
- 1 cup quinoa, rinsed
- 2 cups vegetable broth or water
- 1 tablespoon olive oil
- 1 onion, diced
- 2 cloves garlic, minced
- 1 carrot, diced
- 1 zucchini, diced
- 1 cup diced tomatoes (fresh or canned)
- 1 teaspoon dried oregano
- 1 teaspoon dried basil
- Salt and pepper to taste
- 1 cup shredded cheese (such as cheddar, mozzarella, or feta), divided
- Chopped fresh parsley or basil for garnish (optional)

Instructions:
- Preheat your oven to 375°F (190°C).

- In a medium saucepan, bring the vegetable broth or water to a boil. Add the quinoa, reduce the heat to low, cover, and simmer for about 15 minutes, or until the quinoa is cooked and the liquid is absorbed.

- While the quinoa is cooking, heat the olive oil in a large skillet over medium heat. Add the diced onion and garlic, and cook for 2-3 minutes until softened. Add the diced carrot and zucchini to the skillet, and cook for another 5 minutes until softened.

- Stir in the diced tomatoes, dried oregano, dried basil, salt, and pepper. Cook for 2-3 minutes until the mixture is heated through. In a large mixing bowl, combine the cooked quinoa with the vegetable mixture. Stir in 1/2 cup of shredded cheese until well combined.

- Arrange the halved bell peppers in a baking dish, cut side up. Spoon the quinoa and vegetable mixture into each bell pepper half, pressing down gently to pack the filling.

- Cover the baking dish with aluminum foil and bake in the preheated oven for 25-30 minutes, or until the bell peppers are tender. Remove the foil from the baking dish, sprinkle the remaining 1/2 cup of shredded cheese over the stuffed bell peppers, and return them to the oven. Bake for an additional 5 minutes, or until the cheese is melted and bubbly.

- Remove the stuffed bell peppers from the oven and let them cool for a few minutes. Garnish with chopped fresh parsley or basil, if desired, before serving.

These quinoa-stuffed bell peppers are a nutritious and satisfying option for individuals with ADHD and autism. They're packed with protein, fiber, vitamins, and minerals, and they're easy to customize with your favorite vegetables and cheese. Plus, they make a colorful and flavorful meal that's perfect for lunch or dinner.

35. Spaghetti squash with marinara sauce

Ingredients:

- 1 medium spaghetti squash
- 2 cups marinara sauce (homemade or store-bought)
- Olive oil
- Salt and pepper to taste
- Optional toppings: grated Parmesan cheese, chopped fresh basil, or crushed red pepper flakes

Instructions:

- Preheat your oven to 400°F (200°C).

- Cut the spaghetti squash in half lengthwise and scoop out the seeds with a spoon. Brush the cut sides of the spaghetti squash with olive oil and sprinkle with salt and pepper.

- Place the spaghetti squash halves, cut side down, on a baking sheet lined with parchment paper.

- Roast the spaghetti squash in the preheated oven for 35-45 minutes, or until the flesh is tender and easily pierced with a fork.

- While the spaghetti squash is roasting, heat the marinara sauce in a saucepan over medium heat until warmed through.

- Once the spaghetti squash is cooked, remove it from the oven and let it cool for a few minutes.

- Use a fork to scrape the flesh of the spaghetti squash into strands. The flesh should easily come apart into spaghetti-like strands.

- Divide the spaghetti squash strands among serving plates or bowls. Spoon the warm marinara sauce over the spaghetti squash.

- If desired, sprinkle grated Parmesan cheese, chopped fresh basil, or crushed red pepper flakes over the top for extra flavor. Serve the spaghetti squash with marinara sauce immediately and enjoy!

This spaghetti squash with marinara sauce is a nutritious and satisfying option for individuals with ADHD and autism. It's low in carbs, gluten-free, and packed with vitamins, minerals, and fiber. Plus, it's a delicious alternative to traditional pasta and can be customized with your favorite toppings and herbs for added flavor.

36. Grilled shrimp with asparagus

Ingredients:
- 1 lb large shrimp, peeled and deveined
- 1 lb asparagus spears, trimmed
- 2 tablespoons olive oil
- 2 cloves garlic, minced
- 1 teaspoon lemon zest
- 2 tablespoons lemon juice
- Salt and pepper to taste
- Optional: chopped fresh parsley or cilantro for garnish

Instructions:
- Preheat your grill to medium-high heat.

- In a small bowl, whisk together the olive oil, minced garlic, lemon zest, lemon juice, salt, and pepper to make the marinade.

- Place the shrimp in a large resealable plastic bag or shallow dish. Pour the marinade over the shrimp and toss to coat evenly. Let the shrimp marinate in the refrigerator for 15-30 minutes.

- While the shrimp is marinating, toss the trimmed asparagus spears with a drizzle of olive oil, salt, and pepper.

- Thread the marinated shrimp onto skewers, alternating with the asparagus spears.

- Grill the shrimp and asparagus skewers over medium-high heat for 2-3 minutes per side, or until the shrimp are pink and opaque and the asparagus is tender and slightly charred.

- Remove the skewers from the grill and transfer them to a serving platter. If desired, garnish the grilled shrimp and asparagus with chopped fresh parsley or cilantro.

- Serve the grilled shrimp and asparagus hot, with lemon wedges on the side for squeezing over the top.

This grilled shrimp with asparagus is a nutritious and delicious option for individuals with ADHD and autism. Shrimp is rich in protein and omega-3 fatty acids, while asparagus is packed with vitamins, minerals, and fiber. Plus, grilling adds a smoky flavor to the dish, making it even more flavorful. Enjoy this dish as a main course or as part of a balanced meal.

37. Pork tenderloin with roasted vegetables

Ingredients:
- 1 pork tenderloin (about 1 to 1.5 lbs)
- 2 tablespoons olive oil, divided
- 2 cloves garlic, minced
- 1 teaspoon dried thyme
- 1 teaspoon dried rosemary
- Salt and pepper to taste
- 2 cups assorted vegetables (such as carrots, potatoes, bell peppers, onions, and zucchini), cut into bite-sized pieces
- Optional: fresh herbs (such as parsley or thyme) for garnish

Instructions:
- Preheat your oven to 400°F (200°C).

- In a small bowl, mix together 1 tablespoon of olive oil, minced garlic, dried thyme, dried rosemary, salt, and pepper to make a marinade.

- Place the pork tenderloin in a shallow dish and rub the marinade all over the pork, coating it evenly. Let it marinate for at least 30 minutes, or up to overnight in the refrigerator.

- While the pork is marinating, prepare the vegetables. Place the assorted vegetables on a baking sheet lined with parchment paper. Drizzle with the remaining tablespoon of olive oil, and season with salt and pepper to taste. Toss to coat the vegetables evenly.

- Once the pork has finished marinating, place it on the baking sheet with the vegetables.

- Roast in the preheated oven for 25-30 minutes, or until the pork reaches an internal temperature of 145°F (63°C) and the vegetables are tender and lightly browned, stirring the vegetables halfway through cooking.

- Remove the pork tenderloin from the oven and let it rest for 5-10 minutes before slicing. Slice the pork tenderloin into medallions and serve with the roasted vegetables. Garnish with fresh herbs, if desired, before serving.

This pork tenderloin with roasted vegetables is a nutritious and satisfying option for individuals with ADHD and autism. It's packed with protein, vitamins, and minerals from the pork and vegetables, and it's easy to prepare with minimal fuss. Plus, it's a versatile dish that can be customized with your favorite vegetables and herbs. Enjoy it as a wholesome and flavorful meal any day of the week!

38. Zucchini noodles with pesto

Ingredients:
- 4 medium zucchini
- 1 cup fresh basil leaves, packed
- 1/4 cup pine nuts or walnuts
- 2 cloves garlic
- 1/4 cup grated Parmesan cheese
- 1/4 cup extra virgin olive oil
- Salt and pepper to taste
- Optional toppings: cherry tomatoes, sliced olives, shredded Parmesan cheese, or crushed red pepper flakes

Instructions:
- Using a spiralizer or vegetable peeler, cut the zucchini into noodles or ribbons. Set aside.

- In a food processor or blender, combine the basil leaves, pine nuts or walnuts, garlic, and grated Parmesan cheese. Pulse until finely chopped.

- With the food processor or blender running, slowly drizzle in the olive oil until the pesto is smooth and well combined. Season with salt and pepper to taste.

- In a large skillet, heat a drizzle of olive oil over medium heat. Add the zucchini noodles to the skillet and toss gently for 2-3 minutes, or until heated through and slightly softened.

- Add the pesto to the skillet with the zucchini noodles and toss until the noodles are evenly coated with the pesto sauce.

- Remove the skillet from the heat and divide the zucchini noodles among serving plates or bowls.

- If desired, top the zucchini noodles with cherry tomatoes, sliced olives, shredded Parmesan cheese, or crushed red pepper flakes for extra flavor and texture.

- Serve the zucchini noodles with pesto immediately and enjoy!

This zucchini noodles with pesto is a nutritious and delicious option for individuals with ADHD and autism. It's low in carbs, gluten-free, and packed with vitamins, minerals, and healthy fats. Plus, it's quick and easy to make, making it perfect for a quick and healthy weeknight meal. Feel free to customize the dish with your favorite toppings and herbs for added flavor.

39. Chicken curry with cauliflower rice

Ingredients for Chicken Curry:
- 1 lb boneless, skinless chicken breasts or thighs, cut into bite-sized pieces
- 1 tablespoon olive oil or coconut oil
- 1 onion, diced
- 2 cloves garlic, minced
- 1 tablespoon fresh ginger, minced
- 2 tablespoons curry powder
- 1 teaspoon ground turmeric
- 1 teaspoon ground cumin
- 1 cup chicken broth
- 2 cups cauliflower florets
- 1/2 teaspoon ground coriander
- 1/4 teaspoon cayenne pepper (optional, for heat)
- 1 can (14 oz) coconut milk
- Salt and pepper to taste
- Fresh cilantro for garnish (optional)

Ingredients for Cauliflower Rice:
- 1 head cauliflower
- 1 tablespoon olive oil or coconut oil
- Salt and pepper to taste

Instructions for Chicken Curry:
- In a large skillet or Dutch oven, heat the olive oil over medium heat. Add the diced onion and cook until softened, about 5 minutes.

- Add the minced garlic and ginger to the skillet and cook for another 1-2 minutes, until fragrant. Add the chicken pieces to the skillet and cook until browned on all sides, about 5-7 minutes.

- Stir in the curry powder, ground turmeric, ground cumin, ground coriander, and cayenne pepper (if using). Cook for 1 minute until fragrant. Pour in the coconut milk and chicken broth, stirring to combine. Bring the mixture to a simmer.

- Add the cauliflower florets to the skillet and stir to combine. Cover and simmer for 15-20 minutes, stirring occasionally, until the chicken is cooked through and the cauliflower is tender.

- Season with salt and pepper to taste. If the curry is too thick, you can add more chicken broth or coconut milk to reach your desired consistency. Garnish with fresh cilantro, if desired, before serving.

Instructions for Cauliflower Rice:
- Cut the cauliflower into florets and place them in a food processor. Pulse the cauliflower until it resembles rice-like grains.

- Heat the olive oil or coconut oil in a large skillet over medium heat. Add the cauliflower rice to the skillet and season with salt and pepper to taste. Cook, stirring occasionally, for 5-7 minutes, until the cauliflower is tender but still slightly crisp.

40. Vegetarian chili

Ingredients:
- 1 tablespoon olive oil
- 1 onion, diced
- 2 cloves garlic, minced
- 1 bell pepper, diced
- 1 zucchini, diced
- 1 carrot, diced
- 1 can (14 oz) diced tomatoes
- 1 can (15 oz) kidney beans, drained and rinsed
- 1 can (15 oz) black beans, drained and rinsed
- 1 cup frozen corn kernels
- 1 cup vegetable broth
- 2 tablespoons chili powder
- 1 teaspoon ground cumin
- 1 teaspoon paprika
- 1/2 teaspoon dried oregano
- Salt and pepper to taste
- Optional toppings: shredded cheese, chopped green onions, sour cream, avocado slices, or cilantro

Instructions:
- Heat the olive oil in a large pot over medium heat. Add the diced onion and cook until softened, about 5 minutes.

- Add the minced garlic, diced bell pepper, diced zucchini, and diced carrot to the pot. Cook for another 5 minutes, until the vegetables are tender.

- Stir in the diced tomatoes, kidney beans, black beans, frozen corn kernels, vegetable broth, chili powder, ground cumin, paprika, dried oregano, salt, and pepper.

- Bring the chili to a simmer, then reduce the heat to low. Cover and let it simmer for 20-30 minutes, stirring occasionally, to allow the flavors to meld together.

- Taste and adjust the seasoning as needed. Serve the vegetarian chili hot, topped with your favorite toppings such as shredded cheese, chopped green onions, sour cream, avocado slices, or cilantro.

This vegetarian chili is rich in flavor, protein, and fiber, making it a nutritious and satisfying option for individuals with ADHD and autism. It's easy to make, customizable with your favorite vegetables and toppings, and perfect for a cozy and comforting meal any time of year. Enjoy it on its own or with a side of crusty bread or tortilla chips for dipping.

41. Fresh fruit salad

Ingredients:

- Assorted fresh fruits (such as strawberries, blueberries, grapes, pineapple, kiwi, oranges, and bananas)
- Optional: honey or maple syrup for drizzling
- Optional: chopped mint leaves for garnish

Instructions:

- Wash and prepare the fruits. Cut larger fruits like pineapple and melons into bite-sized pieces. Slice strawberries, kiwi, and bananas.

- Combine the prepared fruits in a large bowl.

- If desired, drizzle honey or maple syrup over the fruit salad for added sweetness. Toss gently to coat.

- Garnish with chopped mint leaves for a refreshing touch.

- Serve the fresh fruit salad immediately, or cover and refrigerate until ready to serve.

Fresh fruit salad is a nutritious and delicious option for individuals with ADHD and autism. It's packed with vitamins, minerals, and antioxidants, and it's naturally sweet and flavorful. Plus, you can customize it with your favorite fruits and toppings for variety. Enjoy it as a refreshing snack or side dish any time of day.

42. Chia pudding with coconut milk

Ingredients:

- 1/4 cup chia seeds
- 1 cup coconut milk (or any other milk of your choice)
- 1 tablespoon maple syrup or honey (optional, for sweetness)
- 1/2 teaspoon vanilla extract (optional, for flavor)
- Fresh fruit, nuts, or seeds for topping (optional)

Instructions:

- In a bowl or jar, combine the chia seeds, coconut milk, maple syrup or honey (if using), and vanilla extract (if using). Stir well to combine.

- Cover the bowl or jar and refrigerate for at least 2 hours, or preferably overnight, to allow the chia seeds to absorb the liquid and thicken.

- After the chia pudding has set, give it a stir to break up any clumps and evenly distribute the seeds.

- If desired, top the chia pudding with fresh fruit, nuts, or seeds for added flavor, texture, and nutrients.

- Serve the chia pudding cold as a nutritious and satisfying breakfast, snack, or dessert.

Chia pudding with coconut milk is a nutritious and delicious option for individuals with ADHD and autism. Chia seeds are rich in fiber, omega-3 fatty acids, protein, and various nutrients, while coconut milk adds creaminess and a subtle tropical flavor. Plus, you can customize the pudding with your favorite toppings and flavors for variety. Enjoy it as a wholesome and flavorful treat any time of day!

43. Banana ice cream

Ingredients:
Ripe bananas

Instructions:

- Peel ripe bananas and cut them into coins or chunks.

- Place the banana pieces in a single layer on a baking sheet lined with parchment paper or a silicone mat.

- Freeze the banana pieces for at least 2 hours, or until they are completely frozen.

- Once the banana pieces are frozen, transfer them to a food processor or high-powered blender.

- Blend the frozen banana pieces until smooth and creamy, scraping down the sides of the food processor or blender as needed. This process may take a few minutes and may require stopping to stir the banana pieces occasionally.

- Once the banana mixture is smooth and creamy, it will resemble soft-serve ice cream.

- Serve the banana ice cream immediately for a soft-serve consistency, or transfer it to a container and freeze for an additional 1-2 hours for a firmer texture.

- Enjoy the banana ice cream plain or with your favorite toppings, such as chopped nuts, fresh fruit, chocolate chips, or a drizzle of honey.

Banana ice cream is a nutritious and delicious option for individuals with ADHD and autism. It's naturally sweet, creamy, and dairy-free, making it suitable for those with dietary restrictions or preferences. Plus, it's a great way to use up ripe bananas and reduce food waste. Enjoy this guilt-free treat as a refreshing dessert or snack any time of day!

44. Dark chocolate covered strawberries

Ingredients:

- Fresh strawberries
- Dark chocolate chips or chopped dark chocolate (at least 70% cocoa)
- Optional: white chocolate chips or chopped white chocolate (for drizzling)

Instructions:
- Wash and dry the strawberries thoroughly. Make sure they are completely dry before dipping them in chocolate to prevent the chocolate from seizing.

- Line a baking sheet with parchment paper or wax paper.

- In a microwave-safe bowl, melt the dark chocolate chips or chopped dark chocolate in 30-second intervals, stirring between each interval, until smooth and melted. Be careful not to overheat the chocolate.

- Hold a strawberry by the stem and dip it into the melted chocolate, swirling to coat about two-thirds of the strawberry.

- Allow any excess chocolate to drip off, then place the chocolate-covered strawberry on the prepared baking sheet.

- Repeat the process with the remaining strawberries.

- If desired, melt the white chocolate chips or chopped white chocolate in a separate microwave-safe bowl and drizzle it over the chocolate-covered strawberries for decoration.

- Place the baking sheet in the refrigerator for about 10-15 minutes to allow the chocolate to set.

- Once the chocolate has hardened, remove the chocolate-covered strawberries from the refrigerator and serve immediately, or store them in an airtight container in the refrigerator until ready to serve.

Dark chocolate covered strawberries are a delicious and indulgent treat that's also relatively healthy. Dark chocolate is rich in antioxidants and lower in sugar compared to milk chocolate, and strawberries are packed with vitamins and minerals. Plus, they're easy to make and perfect for special occasions or as a romantic dessert. Enjoy these decadent treats as a delightful snack or dessert!

45. Baked apples with cinnamon

Ingredients:

- Apples (any variety you prefer)
- Ground cinnamon
- Optional toppings: chopped nuts, raisins, honey, maple syrup, or a sprinkle of brown sugar

Instructions:

- Preheat your oven to 375°F (190°C).

- Wash and core the apples. You can leave the skins on or peel them, depending on your preference.

- Using a paring knife or apple corer, remove the core from the center of each apple, leaving the bottom intact to create a well for the filling.

- Place the cored apples in a baking dish or on a baking sheet lined with parchment paper.
- Sprinkle ground cinnamon generously over each apple, filling the well where the core was removed.

- If desired, fill the center of each apple with optional toppings such as chopped nuts, raisins, honey, maple syrup, or a sprinkle of brown sugar.

- Cover the baking dish with aluminum foil and bake in the preheated oven for 25-30 minutes, or until the apples are tender and can be easily pierced with a fork.

- Remove the foil and continue baking for an additional 5-10 minutes to allow the tops of the apples to brown slightly.

- Once baked, remove the apples from the oven and let them cool for a few minutes before serving.

- Serve the baked apples warm, optionally topped with a scoop of vanilla ice cream or a dollop of whipped cream for an extra treat.

Baked apples with cinnamon are a nutritious and comforting dessert that's perfect for any occasion. They're naturally sweet, fragrant with cinnamon, and wonderfully tender when baked. Plus, you can customize them with your favorite toppings to suit your taste preferences. Enjoy these warm and cozy treats as a satisfying dessert or snack!

46. Coconut macaroons

Ingredients:

- 3 cups shredded coconut (sweetened or unsweetened, depending on your preference)
- 3/4 cup sweetened condensed milk
- 1 teaspoon vanilla extract
- 2 large egg whites
- Pinch of salt

Instructions:

- Preheat your oven to 325°F (160°C). Line a baking sheet with parchment paper or a silicone baking mat.

- In a large mixing bowl, combine the shredded coconut, sweetened condensed milk, and vanilla extract. Stir until well combined.

- In a separate clean bowl, beat the egg whites with a pinch of salt until stiff peaks form.

- Gently fold the beaten egg whites into the coconut mixture until evenly incorporated. Be careful not to deflate the egg whites too much.

- Using a spoon or a small cookie scoop, drop rounded tablespoons of the coconut mixture onto the prepared baking sheet, spacing them about 1 inch apart.

- Bake in the preheated oven for 15-20 minutes, or until the macaroons are golden brown around the edges.

- Remove the macaroons from the oven and let them cool on the baking sheet for a few minutes before transferring them to a wire rack to cool completely.

- Once cooled, the macaroons can be stored in an airtight container at room temperature for several days.

These coconut macaroons are sweet, chewy, and full of coconut flavor. They're a delightful treat for individuals with ADHD and autism, and they're perfect for special occasions or as a sweet snack any time of day. Feel free to customize the recipe by adding chocolate chips, chopped nuts, or other flavorings to suit your taste preferences. Enjoy!

47. Yogurt parfait with granola and fruit

Ingredients:

- Greek yogurt (plain or flavored, depending on your preference)
- Granola (store-bought or homemade)
- Assorted fresh fruits (such as berries, sliced bananas, diced apples, or chopped mango)
- Optional: honey or maple syrup for drizzling
- Optional: shredded coconut, chopped nuts, or seeds for topping

Instructions:

- In a serving glass or bowl, layer Greek yogurt, granola, and fresh fruits.

- Repeat the layers until the glass or bowl is filled, ending with a layer of yogurt on top.

- If desired, drizzle honey or maple syrup over the top layer of yogurt for added sweetness.

- Sprinkle shredded coconut, chopped nuts, or seeds on top for extra flavor and texture.

- Serve the yogurt parfait immediately and enjoy!

Yogurt parfaits with granola and fruit are a nutritious and delicious option for individuals with ADHD and autism. Greek yogurt is rich in protein and probiotics, while granola provides fiber and crunch, and fresh fruits add natural sweetness and vitamins. Plus, you can customize the parfait with your favorite fruits, toppings, and flavors for variety. Enjoy it as a wholesome breakfast, snack, or dessert any time of day!

48. Almond flour brownies

Ingredients:

- 1/2 cup (1 stick) unsalted butter, melted
- 1 cup granulated sugar or coconut sugar
- 2 large eggs
- 1 teaspoon vanilla extract
- 1/2 cup unsweetened cocoa powder
- 1/2 cup almond flour
- 1/4 teaspoon salt
- Optional: chopped nuts, chocolate chips, or shredded coconut for topping

Instructions:

- Preheat your oven to 350°F (175°C). Grease or line an 8x8-inch baking pan with parchment paper.

- In a large mixing bowl, whisk together the melted butter and sugar until well combined.

- Add the eggs and vanilla extract to the bowl, and whisk until smooth and creamy.

- Sift the cocoa powder into the bowl, then add the almond flour and salt. Stir until just combined, being careful not to overmix.

- Pour the brownie batter into the prepared baking pan, spreading it out evenly with a spatula.

- If desired, sprinkle chopped nuts, chocolate chips, or shredded coconut over the top of the batter.

- Bake in the preheated oven for 25-30 minutes, or until a toothpick inserted into the center comes out with a few moist crumbs attached.

- Remove the brownies from the oven and let them cool completely in the pan before slicing and serving.

These almond flour brownies are rich, fudgy, and indulgent, making them a perfect treat for individuals with ADHD and autism. Almond flour adds a nutty flavor and a tender texture to the brownies, while cocoa powder provides rich chocolatey flavor. Plus, they're gluten-free and lower in carbs compared to traditional brownies. Enjoy these delicious brownies as a satisfying dessert or snack!

49. Mango sorbet

Ingredients:
4 ripe mangoes, peeled, pitted, and diced
1/2 cup granulated sugar (adjust to taste depending on the sweetness of the mangoes)
1/4 cup water
1 tablespoon fresh lime or lemon juice (optional, for added brightness)

Instructions:
- Place the diced mangoes in a blender or food processor.

- In a small saucepan, combine the granulated sugar and water. Heat over medium heat, stirring occasionally, until the sugar is completely dissolved. Remove from heat and let the syrup cool slightly.

- Pour the sugar syrup over the diced mangoes in the blender or food processor.

- Add the fresh lime or lemon juice, if using.

- Blend the mixture until smooth and creamy.

- Taste the mango puree and adjust the sweetness or tartness by adding more sugar or lime/lemon juice if needed.

- Transfer the mango puree to a shallow dish or baking pan.

- Cover the dish with plastic wrap and place it in the freezer.

- Freeze the mango puree for at least 4-6 hours, or until firm.

- Once the mango mixture is frozen, remove it from the freezer and let it sit at room temperature for a few minutes to soften slightly.

- Scoop the mango sorbet into bowls or cones and serve immediately.

- Optionally, garnish with fresh mint leaves or slices of mango before serving.

This mango sorbet is a refreshing and dairy-free dessert option for individuals with ADHD and autism. It's naturally sweet, tangy, and bursting with tropical flavor. Plus, it's made with simple ingredients and doesn't require an ice cream maker. Enjoy this cool and refreshing treat on a hot day or anytime you're craving something sweet and fruity!

50. Peanut butter cookies

Ingredients:

- 1 cup peanut butter (creamy or crunchy, depending on your preference)
- 1 cup granulated sugar
- 1 large egg
- 1 teaspoon vanilla extract
- Optional: chocolate chips, chopped nuts, or a sprinkle of sea salt for topping

Instructions:

- Preheat your oven to 350°F (175°C). Line a baking sheet with parchment paper or lightly grease it.

- In a mixing bowl, combine the peanut butter, granulated sugar, egg, and vanilla extract. Stir until the mixture is smooth and well combined.

- If desired, fold in chocolate chips or chopped nuts for extra flavor and texture.

- Using a spoon or cookie scoop, drop rounded tablespoons of dough onto the prepared baking sheet, spacing them about 2 inches apart.

- Flatten each dough ball slightly with a fork, creating a crisscross pattern on top.

- Optionally, sprinkle a pinch of sea salt over each cookie for a sweet and salty flavor contrast.

- Bake the cookies in the preheated oven for 10-12 minutes, or until they are lightly golden brown around the edges.

- Remove the cookies from the oven and let them cool on the baking sheet for a few minutes before transferring them to a wire rack to cool completely.

- Once cooled, the peanut butter cookies can be stored in an airtight container at room temperature for several days.

These peanut butter cookies are soft, chewy, and packed with peanut flavor. They're a comforting and satisfying treat for individuals with ADHD and autism, and they're perfect for sharing with family and friends. Feel free to customize the recipe by adding your favorite mix-ins or toppings. Enjoy these delicious cookies as a snack or dessert any time of day!

51. Sushi rolls with cucumber and avocado

Ingredients:

- Sushi rice (short-grain rice)
- Nori (seaweed) sheets
- Cucumber, julienned into long strips
- Avocado, sliced
- Rice vinegar
- Sugar
- Salt
- Soy sauce, for serving
- Pickled ginger, for serving
- Wasabi, for serving
- Optional: sesame seeds, for garnish

Instructions:

- Cook the sushi rice according to package instructions. Once cooked, transfer the rice to a large bowl and let it cool slightly.

- In a small bowl, mix together rice vinegar, sugar, and salt to make sushi vinegar. Pour the sushi vinegar over the cooked rice and gently fold it in using a spatula or rice paddle until well combined. Let the seasoned rice cool to room temperature.

- Place a sheet of nori shiny side down on a bamboo sushi mat or a clean kitchen towel.
- With damp hands, spread a thin layer of sushi rice evenly over the nori, leaving about 1 inch of space at the top edge.

- Arrange julienned cucumber and sliced avocado horizontally across the center of the rice-covered nori sheet.

- Using the bamboo sushi mat or kitchen towel, tightly roll the sushi away from you, using gentle pressure to shape it into a compact cylinder.

- Once rolled, seal the edge of the nori sheet by lightly wetting it with water.

- Using a sharp knife, carefully slice the sushi roll into individual pieces, wiping the knife clean between cuts.

- Arrange the sushi rolls on a serving platter, sprinkle with sesame seeds if desired, and serve with soy sauce, pickled ginger, and wasabi on the side.

These homemade sushi rolls with cucumber and avocado are fresh, flavorful, and nutritious. They're a great option for individuals with ADHD and autism, as they provide a sensory-rich experience and can be customized to suit personal preferences. Enjoy them as a delicious and satisfying meal or snack!

52. Chicken tikka masala with basmati rice

Ingredients for Chicken Tikka:
* 1 lb boneless, skinless chicken breasts
or thighs, cut into bite-sized pieces
* 1 cup plain yogurt
* 2 tablespoons lemon juice
* 2 teaspoons ground cumin
* 2 teaspoons ground paprika
* 1 teaspoon ground turmeric
* 1 teaspoon ground coriander
* 1 teaspoon garam masala
* 1 teaspoon salt
* 1/2 teaspoon black pepper
* 2 cloves garlic, minced
* 1 tablespoon grated ginger
* 2 tablespoons vegetable oil,
for grilling or broiling

Ingredients for Basmati Rice:
* 1 cup basmati rice
* 1 3/4 cups water
* 1 tablespoon butter or ghee
* Salt to taste

Ingredients for Tikka Masala Sauce:

2 tablespoons vegetable oil or ghee
* 1 onion, finely chopped
* 2 cloves garlic, minced
* 1 tablespoon grated ginger
* 1 tablespoon tomato paste
* 1 can (14 oz) crushed tomatoes
* 1 cup heavy cream or coconut milk
* 1 teaspoon ground cumin
* 1 teaspoon ground coriander
* 1 teaspoon garam masala
* 1/2 teaspoon ground turmeric
* Salt and pepper to taste
* Fresh cilantro, chopped, for garnish

Instructions:
* In a large bowl, combine yogurt, lemon juice, ground cumin, paprika, turmeric, coriander, garam masala, salt, pepper, minced garlic, and grated ginger. Mix well. Add the chicken pieces to the marinade and coat them evenly. Cover the bowl and refrigerate for at least 1 hour, or overnight for best results.

* Preheat your grill or broiler. Thread the marinated chicken pieces onto skewers and grill or broil until cooked through and slightly charred, about 10-12 minutes, turning occasionally.

* In a large skillet, heat vegetable oil or ghee over medium heat. Add chopped onion and cook until softened, about 5 minutes. Add minced garlic and grated ginger to the skillet and cook for another 1-2 minutes, until fragrant.

* Stir in tomato paste and cook for 1 minute. Add crushed tomatoes, ground cumin, ground coriander, garam masala, ground turmeric, salt, and pepper to the skillet. Bring to a simmer and cook for 10-15 minutes, stirring occasionally, until the sauce has thickened slightly.

- Stir in heavy cream or coconut milk and cooked chicken tikka pieces. Simmer for an additional 5 minutes to heat through.

- While the sauce is simmering, rinse basmati rice under cold water until the water runs clear. Drain well.

- In a medium saucepan, combine basmati rice, water, butter or ghee, and salt. Bring to a boil, then reduce the heat to low, cover, and simmer for 15-20 minutes, or until the rice is tender and the water is absorbed. Remove from heat and let it sit, covered, for 5 minutes.

- Fluff the cooked rice with a fork and serve hot with chicken tikka masala. Garnish the chicken tikka masala with chopped fresh cilantro before serving.

This chicken tikka masala with basmati rice is a flavorful and comforting dish that's perfect for individuals with ADHD and autism. It's rich in spices and aromatics, providing a sensory-rich experience, and it's served with fluffy basmati rice for a satisfying meal. Enjoy it as a delicious and nourishing dinner option!

53. Beef pho with rice noodles

Ingredients for Beef Broth:
2 lbs beef bones (such as marrow bones or oxtails)
1 onion, halved
1 piece (about 2 inches) fresh ginger, halved lengthwise
2 cinnamon sticks
4 star anise
4 cloves
1 cardamom pod
1 tablespoon coriander seeds
1 teaspoon fennel seeds
1 tablespoon salt
1 tablespoon sugar
Water

Ingredients for Pho Bowl:
- 8 oz dried rice noodles (banh pho)
- 1 lb beef sirloin or flank steak, thinly sliced
- Garnishes: thinly sliced onion, chopped green onions, fresh cilantro, Thai basil leaves, bean sprouts, lime wedges, thinly sliced jalapeno or Thai chili peppers
- Hoisin sauce and sriracha sauce, for serving

Instructions:
- To make the beef broth, place the beef bones in a large pot and cover with water. Bring to a boil, then reduce the heat to low and simmer for about 10 minutes. Drain the bones and rinse them under cold water to remove any impurities.

- Return the bones to the pot and add fresh water to cover. Add the halved onion and ginger, cinnamon sticks, star anise, cloves, cardamom pod, coriander seeds, fennel seeds, salt, and sugar.

- Bring the broth to a boil, then reduce the heat to low and simmer, uncovered, for at least 1 hour, but preferably 2-3 hours, skimming off any foam that rises to the surface.

- While the broth is simmering, prepare the rice noodles according to the package instructions. Drain and set aside.

- Once the broth is done simmering, strain it through a fine-mesh sieve or cheesecloth-lined colander into a clean pot. Discard the solids.

- Bring the strained broth back to a simmer. Taste and adjust the seasoning with more salt and sugar if needed.

- To serve, divide the cooked rice noodles among serving bowls. Top with thinly sliced beef sirloin or flank steak.

- Ladle the hot broth over the noodles and beef, ensuring that the beef is submerged in the hot broth to cook it.

- Serve the beef pho hot, accompanied by garnishes such as thinly sliced onion, chopped green onions, fresh cilantro, Thai basil leaves, bean sprouts, lime wedges, and thinly sliced jalapeno or Thai chili peppers.

- Allow diners to customize their bowls of pho with hoisin sauce, sriracha sauce, and additional garnishes to taste.

Beef pho with rice noodles is a comforting and aromatic dish that's perfect for individuals with ADHD and autism. It's rich in flavor, texture, and aroma, providing a sensory-rich experience. Plus, it's customizable with a variety of fresh herbs, vegetables, and condiments, allowing for individual preferences. Enjoy this delicious and nourishing Vietnamese soup as a comforting meal any time of day!

54. Vegetable pad thai

Ingredients for Pad Thai Sauce:
- 3 tablespoons soy sauce
- 2 tablespoons tamarind paste
- 2 tablespoons brown sugar
- 1 tablespoon fish sauce

(optional, omit for vegetarian/vegan)
- 1 tablespoon lime juice
- 1 teaspoon sriracha sauce

or chili flakes (adjust to taste)

Instructions:
- In a small bowl, whisk together the

soy sauce, tamarind paste, brown
sugar, fish sauce (if using), lime
juice, and sriracha sauce or
chili flakes until well combined. Set aside.

Ingredients for Vegetable Pad Thai:
8 oz pad Thai rice noodles
2 tablespoons vegetable oil
3 cloves garlic, minced
1 small onion, thinly sliced
2 carrots, julienned
1 red bell pepper, thinly sliced
1 cup broccoli florets
1 cup bean sprouts
1/2 cup sliced green onions
1/4 cup chopped cilantro
1/4 cup chopped peanuts (optional, for garnish)
Lime wedges, for serving

- Cook the pad Thai rice noodles according to the package instructions. Drain and set aside. Heat the vegetable oil in a large skillet or wok over medium-high heat. Add the minced garlic and sliced onion, and cook for 1-2 minutes until fragrant.

- Add the julienned carrots, sliced red bell pepper, and broccoli florets to the skillet. Stir-fry for 3-4 minutes until the vegetables are tender-crisp.

- Push the vegetables to one side of the skillet and crack the eggs into the empty space. Scramble the eggs until cooked through, then mix them with the vegetables.

- Add the cooked rice noodles and pad Thai sauce to the skillet. Toss everything together until well combined and heated through.

- Stir in the bean sprouts, sliced green onions, and chopped cilantro. Cook for another 1-2 minutes until the bean sprouts are slightly wilted.

- Remove the skillet from heat and transfer the vegetable pad Thai to serving plates. Garnish with chopped peanuts (if using) and serve hot with lime wedges on the side.

This vegetable pad Thai is a flavorful and satisfying dish that's perfect for individuals with ADHD and autism. It's packed with a variety of colorful vegetables, providing essential nutrients and textures. Plus, it's customizable to suit personal preferences, so feel free to adjust the ingredients and spice level as needed. Enjoy this delicious and nutritious Thai-inspired dish as a satisfying meal any time of day!

55. Falafel with tahini sauce

Ingredients for Falafel:
- 1 can (15 oz) chickpeas, drained and rinsed
- 1/2 small onion, roughly chopped
- 2 cloves garlic, minced
- 1/4 cup fresh parsley leaves
- 1/4 cup fresh cilantro leaves
- 1 teaspoon ground cumin
- 1 teaspoon ground coriander
- 1/4 teaspoon cayenne pepper (optional, for heat)
- 1/2 teaspoon salt
- 1/4 teaspoon black pepper
- 1 tablespoon chickpea flour or all-purpose flour
- 1 teaspoon baking powder
- Vegetable oil, for frying

Ingredients for Tahini Sauce:
- 1/4 cup tahini (sesame seed paste)
- 2 tablespoons lemon juice
- 2 tablespoons water
- 1 clove garlic, minced
- Salt, to taste

Instructions:
- In a food processor, combine the drained and rinsed chickpeas, chopped onion, minced garlic, parsley, cilantro, ground cumin, ground coriander, cayenne pepper (if using), salt, and black pepper. Pulse until the mixture is coarsely ground and holds together when pressed.

- Transfer the falafel mixture to a mixing bowl. Stir in the chickpea flour or all-purpose flour and baking powder until well combined. The mixture should be thick and hold together easily. If it's too dry, add a little water; if it's too wet, add a little more flour.

- Shape the falafel mixture into small balls or patties, about 1 1/2 inches in diameter.

- In a large skillet, heat vegetable oil over medium heat until hot but not smoking. Carefully add the shaped falafel to the skillet in batches, making sure not to overcrowd the pan.

- Fry the falafel for 3-4 minutes on each side, or until golden brown and crispy. Use a slotted spoon to transfer the cooked falafel to a paper towel-lined plate to drain excess oil.

- To make the tahini sauce, whisk together tahini, lemon juice, water, minced garlic, and salt in a small bowl until smooth and creamy. Adjust the consistency with more water if needed. Serve the falafel hot with tahini sauce drizzled on top or on the side for dipping.

This falafel with tahini sauce is a flavorful and satisfying dish that's perfect for individuals with ADHD and autism. It's packed with plant-based protein, fiber, and essential nutrients, making it a nutritious option. Plus, it's customizable with your favorite toppings and condiments. Enjoy this delicious and nutritious Middle Eastern-inspired dish as a satisfying meal any time of day!

56. Greek salad with olives and feta

Ingredients for Greek Salad:
- 4 cups chopped Romaine lettuce or mixed salad greens
- 1 cucumber, diced
- 1 bell pepper (red, yellow, or green), diced
- 1 cup cherry tomatoes, halved
- 1/2 red onion, thinly sliced
- 1/2 cup Kalamata olives, pitted
- 1/2 cup crumbled feta cheese
- Fresh parsley or oregano leaves, chopped (optional, for garnish)

Ingredients for Greek Salad Dressing:
- 1/4 cup extra virgin olive oil
- 2 tablespoons red wine vinegar or lemon juice
- 1 clove garlic, minced
- 1 teaspoon dried oregano
- Salt and black pepper, to taste

Instructions:
- In a large salad bowl, combine the chopped Romaine lettuce or mixed salad greens, diced cucumber, diced bell pepper, halved cherry tomatoes, thinly sliced red onion, and pitted Kalamata olives.

- In a small bowl, whisk together the extra virgin olive oil, red wine vinegar or lemon juice, minced garlic, dried oregano, salt, and black pepper to make the Greek salad dressing.

- Pour the dressing over the salad ingredients in the bowl and toss until evenly coated.

- Add the crumbled feta cheese to the salad and gently toss to combine.

- Taste and adjust the seasoning with more salt, pepper, or vinegar if needed.

- Garnish the Greek salad with chopped fresh parsley or oregano leaves, if desired. Serve the Greek salad immediately as a side dish or as a light and refreshing meal on its own.

This Greek salad with olives and feta is a flavorful and nutritious dish that's perfect for individuals with ADHD and autism. It's packed with colorful vegetables, briny olives, tangy feta cheese, and a zesty dressing, providing a sensory-rich experience. Plus, it's easy to customize with your favorite salad ingredients and toppings. Enjoy this delicious and refreshing Mediterranean-inspired salad as a satisfying meal any time of day!

57. Tacos with grilled fish

Ingredients for Grilled Fish:
- 1 lb firm white fish fillets
(such as tilapia, cod, or mahi-mahi)
- 2 tablespoons olive oil
- 1 tablespoon lime juice
- 1 teaspoon ground cumin
- 1 teaspoon chili powder
- 1/2 teaspoon garlic powder
- 1/2 teaspoon paprika
- Salt and black pepper, to taste

Ingredients for Tacos:
8 small corn or flour tortillas
Shredded lettuce or cabbage
Diced tomatoes
Sliced avocado
Chopped cilantro
Lime wedges
Optional toppings: salsa, sour cream, diced onions, hot sauce=

Instructions:
- In a shallow dish, whisk together olive oil, lime juice, ground cumin, chili powder, garlic powder, paprika, salt, and black pepper to make the marinade for the fish.

- Place the fish fillets in the marinade, turning to coat evenly. Cover and refrigerate for at least 30 minutes, or up to 2 hours. Preheat your grill or grill pan to medium-high heat. Brush the grill grates with oil to prevent sticking.

- Remove the fish fillets from the marinade and shake off any excess. Grill the fish for 3-4 minutes per side, or until cooked through and lightly charred. The cooking time will depend on the thickness of the fish fillets.

- Once cooked, transfer the grilled fish to a plate and flake it into bite-sized pieces with a fork.

- Warm the tortillas on the grill for 30 seconds to 1 minute per side, or until lightly charred and pliable. To assemble the tacos, fill each warm tortilla with shredded lettuce or cabbage, diced tomatoes, sliced avocado, and grilled fish pieces.

- Garnish the tacos with chopped cilantro and serve with lime wedges on the side. Offer optional toppings such as salsa, sour cream, diced onions, and hot sauce for diners to customize their tacos to taste.

These tacos with grilled fish are a flavorful and nutritious dish that's perfect for individuals with ADHD and autism. The grilled fish provides a good source of protein and healthy fats, while the fresh vegetables add crunch and texture. Plus, they're customizable with your favorite taco toppings and sauces. Enjoy these delicious and satisfying tacos as a tasty meal any time of day!

58. Italian minestrone soup

Ingredients:
- 2 tablespoons olive oil
- 1 onion, diced
- 2 carrots, diced
- 2 celery stalks, diced
- 3 cloves garlic, minced
- 1 can (14 oz) diced tomatoes
- 6 cups vegetable or chicken broth
- 1 can (14 oz) cannellini beans, drained and rinsed
- 1 cup chopped green beans
- 1 cup chopped zucchini
- 1 cup chopped cabbage
- 1 cup small pasta (such as ditalini or elbow macaroni)
- 2 teaspoons dried Italian seasoning
- Salt and black pepper, to taste
- Fresh basil leaves, chopped, for garnish
- Grated Parmesan cheese, for serving (optional)
-

Instructions:
- Heat olive oil in a large pot or Dutch oven over medium heat. Add diced onion, carrots, and celery, and cook for 5-7 minutes until softened.

- Add minced garlic to the pot and cook for an additional 1-2 minutes until fragrant.

- Stir in diced tomatoes and cook for another 2-3 minutes.

- Pour in vegetable or chicken broth and bring the soup to a simmer.

- Add drained and rinsed cannellini beans, chopped green beans, chopped zucchini, chopped cabbage, and dried Italian seasoning to the pot. Stir to combine.

- Simmer the soup uncovered for 15-20 minutes until the vegetables are tender.

- Add small pasta to the pot and continue to simmer for an additional 10-12 minutes until the pasta is cooked al dente.

- Season the minestrone soup with salt and black pepper to taste.

- Ladle the soup into bowls and garnish with chopped fresh basil leaves. Serve the Italian minestrone soup hot, with grated Parmesan cheese on the side for sprinkling over the top if desired.

This Italian minestrone soup is a flavorful and nutritious dish that's perfect for individuals with ADHD and autism. It's packed with a variety of vegetables, beans, and pasta, providing essential nutrients and textures. Plus, it's easy to customize with your favorite ingredients and seasonings. Enjoy this delicious and comforting soup as a satisfying meal any time of day!

59. Spanish paella with seafood

Ingredients:

- 4 cups seafood or chicken broth
- 1 teaspoon smoked paprika
- 1/2 teaspoon saffron threads (optional)
- Salt and black pepper, to taste
- 1/2 cup frozen peas
- Lemon wedges, for serving
- Fresh parsley, chopped, for garnish
- 1 lb mixed seafood (such as shrimp, mussels, clams, and squid), cleaned and deveined
- 2 tablespoons olive oil
- 1 onion, diced
- 2 cloves garlic, minced
- 1 bell pepper (red, yellow, or green), diced
- 1 tomato, diced
- 1 1/2 cups Arborio rice or Spanish short-grain rice (Bomba rice)

Instructions:

- Heat olive oil in a large paella pan or skillet over medium heat. Add diced onion and cook for 3-4 minutes until softened.

- Add minced garlic and diced bell pepper to the pan and cook for another 2-3 minutes until fragrant. Stir in diced tomato and cook for 2-3 minutes until softened.

- Add Arborio rice or Spanish short-grain rice to the pan and cook for 1-2 minutes, stirring constantly, until the rice is coated with oil and lightly toasted. Pour seafood or chicken broth into the pan and bring the liquid to a simmer.

- Add smoked paprika and saffron threads (if using) to the pan. Season with salt and black pepper to taste. Arrange the mixed seafood evenly on top of the rice in the pan.

- Cover the pan with a lid or aluminum foil and simmer for 15-20 minutes until the rice is cooked and the seafood is cooked through. During the last 5 minutes of cooking, sprinkle frozen peas over the top of the paella and cover the pan again to cook the peas.

- Once the paella is done cooking, remove the lid or foil and let it rest for a few minutes. Garnish the paella with chopped fresh parsley and serve hot with lemon wedges on the side.

This Spanish paella with seafood is a delicious and satisfying dish that's perfect for individuals with ADHD and autism. It's packed with a variety of seafood, aromatic spices, and flavorful rice, providing a sensory-rich experience. Plus, it's a one-pan meal that's easy to make and perfect for sharing with family and friends. Enjoy this flavorful and aromatic Spanish dish as a special meal any time of day!

60. Moroccan chickpea stew

Ingredients:

- 2 tablespoons olive oil
- 1 onion, diced
- 2 cloves garlic, minced
- 1 bell pepper

(red, yellow, or green), diced

- 2 carrots, diced
- 2 teaspoons ground cumin
- 1 teaspoon ground coriander
- 1 teaspoon ground turmeric
- 1/2 teaspoon ground cinnamon
- 1/4 teaspoon cayenne pepper (optional, for heat)

- 1 can (14 oz) diced tomatoes
- 2 cups vegetable or chicken broth
- 2 cans (15 oz each) chickpeas, drained and rinsed
- 1/2 cup raisins or chopped dried apricots
- 1/4 cup chopped fresh cilantro or parsley
- Salt and black pepper, to taste
- Cooked couscous or rice, for serving
- Optional toppings: chopped fresh cilantro, chopped nuts, Greek yogurt

Instructions:

- Heat olive oil in a large pot or Dutch oven over medium heat. Add diced onion and cook for 3-4 minutes until softened.

- Add minced garlic, diced bell pepper, and diced carrots to the pot. Cook for another 4-5 minutes until the vegetables are slightly softened.

- Stir in ground cumin, ground coriander, ground turmeric, ground cinnamon, and cayenne pepper (if using). Cook for 1-2 minutes until fragrant.

- Add diced tomatoes and vegetable or chicken broth to the pot. Bring the liquid to a simmer.

- Stir in drained and rinsed chickpeas and raisins or chopped dried apricots. Cover the pot and simmer for 15-20 minutes, stirring occasionally, until the flavors are well blended and the stew has thickened slightly.

- Season the Moroccan chickpea stew with salt and black pepper to taste. Stir in chopped fresh cilantro or parsley just before serving.

- Serve the Moroccan chickpea stew hot over cooked couscous or rice. Garnish with chopped fresh cilantro, chopped nuts, and a dollop of Greek yogurt if desired.

This Moroccan chickpea stew is a flavorful and satisfying dish that's perfect for individuals with ADHD and autism. It's packed with protein-rich chickpeas, aromatic spices, and sweet dried fruit, providing a sensory-rich experience. Plus, it's easy to make and perfect for meal prep. Enjoy this delicious and nutritious Moroccan-inspired stew as a comforting meal any time of day!

61. Stuffed mushrooms

Ingredients:
- 12 large mushrooms, cleaned and stems removed
- 1 tablespoon olive oil
- 2 cloves garlic, minced
- 1/4 cup finely diced onion
- 1/4 cup breadcrumbs (plain or seasoned)
- 1/4 cup grated Parmesan cheese
- 2 tablespoons chopped fresh parsley
- Salt and black pepper, to taste
- Optional: additional grated cheese for topping

Instructions:
- Preheat your oven to 375°F (190°C). Line a baking sheet with parchment paper or lightly grease it with olive oil.

- In a skillet, heat olive oil over medium heat. Add minced garlic and diced onion, and cook for 2-3 minutes until softened and fragrant.

- Chop the mushroom stems finely and add them to the skillet. Cook for another 3-4 minutes until the mushrooms are tender and any excess moisture has evaporated.

- Remove the skillet from heat and transfer the cooked mushroom mixture to a mixing bowl.

- Add breadcrumbs, grated Parmesan cheese, chopped fresh parsley, salt, and black pepper to the bowl. Mix everything together until well combined.

- Take each mushroom cap and spoon a generous amount of the filling mixture into it, pressing gently to pack it in.

- Place the stuffed mushrooms on the prepared baking sheet, evenly spaced apart. If desired, sprinkle additional grated cheese on top of each stuffed mushroom.

- Bake in the preheated oven for 15-20 minutes, or until the mushrooms are tender and the filling is golden brown and slightly crispy on top. Remove the stuffed mushrooms from the oven and let them cool slightly before serving.

These stuffed mushrooms are a flavorful and satisfying dish that's perfect for individuals with ADHD and autism. They're easy to make, packed with savory flavors, and can be customized with your favorite ingredients. Enjoy them as a delicious appetizer, side dish, or even as a light meal!

62. Lentil burgers

Ingredients:

- 1 cup dried lentils
- 2 1/2 cups water or vegetable broth
- 1 tablespoon olive oil
- 1 onion, finely chopped
- 2 cloves garlic, minced
- 1 carrot, grated
- 1/2 cup breadcrumbs
- 1 teaspoon ground cumin
- 1 teaspoon smoked paprika
- 1/2 teaspoon ground coriander
- Salt and black pepper, to taste
- Optional toppings: lettuce, tomato slices, onion slices, avocado, cheese slices, condiments (ketchup, mustard, mayonnaise), whole grain burger buns
- 1/4 cup chopped fresh parsley or cilantro

Instructions:

- Rinse the lentils under cold water and drain them.

- In a medium saucepan, combine the rinsed lentils and water or vegetable broth. Bring to a boil, then reduce the heat to low and simmer for 20-25 minutes, or until the lentils are tender but not mushy. Drain any excess liquid and set aside to cool slightly.

- In a skillet, heat olive oil over medium heat. Add chopped onion and cook for 3-4 minutes until softened. Add minced garlic and grated carrot, and cook for another 2-3 minutes until fragrant.

- In a large mixing bowl, combine the cooked lentils, sautéed onion mixture, breadcrumbs, chopped fresh parsley or cilantro, ground cumin, smoked paprika, ground coriander, salt, and black pepper. Mix everything together until well combined.

- Using your hands, shape the lentil mixture into burger patties of desired size and thickness. Heat a skillet or grill pan over medium-high heat. Add a little olive oil to coat the surface.

- Cook the lentil burgers for 4-5 minutes on each side, or until golden brown and crispy on the outside.

- Once cooked, assemble the lentil burgers with your favorite toppings on whole grain burger buns. Serve the lentil burgers hot and enjoy!

These lentil burgers are a flavorful and satisfying dish that's perfect for individuals with ADHD and autism. They're packed with plant-based protein, fiber, and essential nutrients, making them a nutritious option. Plus, they're versatile and can be customized with your favorite toppings and condiments. Enjoy these delicious and hearty lentil burgers as a tasty meal any time of day!

63. Eggplant parmesan

Ingredients:

- 2 medium eggplants
- Salt
- 2 cups breadcrumbs (plain or seasoned)
- 1 cup grated Parmesan cheese
- Olive oil, for frying
- 2 cups marinara sauce
- 2 cups shredded mozzarella cheese
- Fresh basil leaves, chopped, for garnish (optional)
- 2 eggs, beaten

Instructions:

- Preheat your oven to 375°F (190°C). Grease a baking dish with olive oil or non-stick cooking spray.

- Peel the eggplants (optional) and slice them into rounds, about 1/4 inch thick. Place the eggplant slices in a colander and sprinkle them with salt. Let them sit for 30 minutes to release excess moisture.

- In a shallow dish, combine breadcrumbs and grated Parmesan cheese. Dip each eggplant slice into the beaten eggs, then coat them in the breadcrumb mixture, pressing gently to adhere.

- Heat olive oil in a large skillet over medium heat. Fry the breaded eggplant slices in batches until golden brown and crispy on both sides, about 3-4 minutes per side. Add more oil as needed.

- Transfer the fried eggplant slices to a plate lined with paper towels to drain excess oil. Spread a thin layer of marinara sauce on the bottom of the prepared baking dish. Arrange a layer of fried eggplant slices on top of the sauce.

- Spoon more marinara sauce over the eggplant slices, then sprinkle shredded mozzarella cheese on top. Repeat the layers until all the eggplant slices are used, finishing with a layer of marinara sauce and shredded mozzarella cheese on top.

- Cover the baking dish with aluminum foil and bake in the preheated oven for 25-30 minutes, or until the cheese is melted and bubbly.

- Remove the foil and bake for an additional 5-10 minutes, or until the cheese is golden brown and slightly crispy on top. Remove the eggplant Parmesan from the oven and let it cool for a few minutes before serving. Garnish with chopped fresh basil leaves, if desired, and serve hot.

This eggplant Parmesan is a flavorful and comforting dish that's perfect for individuals with ADHD and autism. It's packed with layers of crispy fried eggplant, savory marinara sauce, and gooey melted cheese, providing a sensory-rich experience. Plus, it's a versatile dish that can be served as a main course or as a side dish alongside pasta or salad. Enjoy this delicious and satisfying Italian classic as a special meal any time of day!

64. Tofu stir-fry

Ingredients:

- 2 cloves garlic, minced
- 1 tablespoon minced ginger
- 1 bell pepper, thinly sliced
- 1 carrot, thinly sliced
- 1 cup broccoli florets
- 1 cup sliced mushrooms
- 2 green onions, sliced
- Cooked rice or noodles, for serving
- 14 oz (400g) firm tofu, pressed and cubed
- 2 tablespoons soy sauce or tamari
- 2 tablespoons rice vinegar or apple cider vinegar
- 1 tablespoon sesame oil
- 1 tablespoon cornstarch
- 2 tablespoons vegetable oil

Instructions:

- In a bowl, whisk together soy sauce, rice vinegar, sesame oil, and cornstarch to make the sauce. Set aside.

- Heat vegetable oil in a large skillet or wok over medium-high heat. Add cubed tofu and cook until golden brown and crispy on all sides, about 5-7 minutes. Remove tofu from the skillet and set aside.

- In the same skillet, add minced garlic and minced ginger. Cook for 1-2 minutes until fragrant.

- Add sliced bell pepper, carrot, broccoli florets, and sliced mushrooms to the skillet. Stir-fry for 5-7 minutes until the vegetables are tender-crisp.

- Return the cooked tofu to the skillet. Pour the sauce over the tofu and vegetables. Stir well to coat everything evenly.

- Cook for another 2-3 minutes until the sauce thickens and coats the tofu and vegetables.
- Remove the skillet from heat and stir in sliced green onions . Serve the tofu stir-fry hot over cooked rice or noodles.

This tofu stir-fry is a delicious and nutritious dish that's perfect for individuals with ADHD and autism. It's packed with protein-rich tofu, colorful vegetables, and a flavorful sauce, providing a sensory-rich experience. Plus, it's versatile and can be customized with your favorite vegetables and seasonings. Enjoy this delicious and satisfying stir-fry as a quick and easy meal any time of day!

65. Vegetable curry

Ingredients:

- 2 tablespoons vegetable oil
- 1 onion, diced
- 2 cloves garlic, minced
- 1 tablespoon minced ginger
- 2 tablespoons curry powder
- 1 teaspoon ground cumin
- 1 teaspoon ground coriander
- 1/2 teaspoon turmeric powder
- 1/4 teaspoon cayenne pepper

(optional, for heat)

- 1 can (14 oz) diced tomatoes
- 1 can (14 oz) coconut milk
- 2 cups chopped mixed vegetables (such as carrots, bell peppers, zucchini, cauliflower, and peas)
- Salt and black pepper, to taste
- Fresh cilantro, chopped, for garnish
- Cooked rice or naan bread, for serving

Instructions:

- Heat vegetable oil in a large skillet or pot over medium heat. Add diced onion and cook for 3-4 minutes until softened.

- Add minced garlic and minced ginger to the skillet. Cook for another 1-2 minutes until fragrant.

- Stir in curry powder, ground cumin, ground coriander, turmeric powder, and cayenne pepper (if using). Cook for 1-2 minutes until the spices are toasted and fragrant.

- Add diced tomatoes (with their juices) to the skillet. Cook for 5-6 minutes, stirring occasionally, until the tomatoes break down and form a thick sauce. Pour in coconut milk and stir to combine. Bring the mixture to a simmer.

- Add chopped mixed vegetables to the skillet. Stir well to coat them in the curry sauce. Cover the skillet and simmer for 15-20 minutes, or until the vegetables are tender.

- Season the vegetable curry with salt and black pepper to taste. Serve the vegetable curry hot over cooked rice or with naan bread. Garnish with chopped fresh cilantro before serving.

This vegetable curry is a flavorful and satisfying dish that's packed with colorful vegetables and aromatic spices, providing a sensory-rich experience. Plus, it's versatile and can be customized with your favorite vegetables and spice levels. Enjoy this delicious and nutritious curry as a comforting meal any time of day!

66. Chickpea salad sandwich

Ingredients:

- 1 can (15 oz) chickpeas, drained and rinsed
- 1/4 cup mayonnaise or vegan mayonnaise
- 1 tablespoon Dijon mustard
- 1 tablespoon lemon juice
- 1/4 cup finely chopped celery
- 1/4 cup finely chopped red onion
- 2 tablespoons chopped fresh parsley or cilantro
- Salt and black pepper, to taste
- Sandwich bread or rolls
- Lettuce leaves, tomato slices, avocado slices (optional, for serving)

Instructions:

- In a mixing bowl, mash the chickpeas with a fork or potato masher until they reach your desired consistency (some prefer chunky, while others prefer smoother).

- Add mayonnaise, Dijon mustard, and lemon juice to the mashed chickpeas. Stir until well combined.

- Add finely chopped celery, red onion, and chopped fresh parsley or cilantro to the bowl. Mix everything together until evenly distributed.

- Season the chickpea salad with salt and black pepper to taste. Adjust seasoning if needed.

- Spread the chickpea salad onto sandwich bread or rolls. Add lettuce leaves, tomato slices, and avocado slices if desired.

- Top with another slice of bread or roll to make a sandwich.

- Slice the sandwiches in half and serve immediately, or wrap them tightly in plastic wrap or parchment paper for later.

These chickpea salad sandwiches are a flavorful and satisfying dish that's perfect for individuals with ADHD and autism. They're packed with protein-rich chickpeas, crunchy vegetables, and creamy dressing, providing a sensory-rich experience. Plus, they're easy to customize with your favorite toppings and can be made ahead for quick and convenient meals. Enjoy these delicious and nutritious sandwiches as a tasty lunch or dinner option!

67. Spinach and ricotta stuffed shells

Ingredients:

- 20 jumbo pasta shells
- 2 cups ricotta cheese
- 1 cup shredded mozzarella cheese
- 1/2 cup grated Parmesan cheese
- 1 egg
- 1 teaspoon garlic powder
- 1 teaspoon dried basil
- 1 teaspoon dried oregano
- Salt and black pepper, to taste
- 2 cups fresh spinach, chopped
- 2 cups marinara sauce
- Fresh basil leaves, chopped, for garnish (optional)

Instructions:

- Preheat your oven to 350°F (175°C). Grease a 9x13 inch baking dish with non-stick cooking spray.

- Cook the jumbo pasta shells according to the package instructions until al dente. Drain and set aside to cool.

- In a large mixing bowl, combine ricotta cheese, shredded mozzarella cheese, grated Parmesan cheese, egg, garlic powder, dried basil, dried oregano, salt, and black pepper. Mix until well combined.

- Stir in chopped fresh spinach until evenly distributed throughout the cheese mixture. Spread 1 cup of marinara sauce evenly over the bottom of the prepared baking dish.

- Stuff each cooked pasta shell with a generous spoonful of the spinach and ricotta mixture. Place the stuffed shells in the baking dish, arranging them in a single layer.

- Pour the remaining marinara sauce over the stuffed shells, covering them completely. Cover the baking dish with aluminum foil and bake in the preheated oven for 25-30 minutes, or until the sauce is bubbly and the cheese is melted.

- Remove the foil and bake for an additional 5-10 minutes, or until the cheese is golden brown and slightly crispy on top.

- Remove the stuffed shells from the oven and let them cool for a few minutes before serving. Garnish with chopped fresh basil leaves, if desired, and serve hot.

These spinach and ricotta stuffed shells are a flavorful and satisfying dish that's perfect for individuals with ADHD and autism. They're packed with creamy ricotta cheese, nutritious spinach, and aromatic herbs, providing a sensory-rich experience. Plus, they're easy to make and perfect for sharing with family and friends. Enjoy this delicious and comforting pasta dish as a special meal any time of day!

68. Black bean and quinoa tacos

Ingredients:

- 1 cup quinoa, rinsed
- 2 cups water or vegetable broth
- 1 can (15 oz) black beans, drained and rinsed
- 1 tablespoon olive oil
- 1 small onion, diced
- 2 cloves garlic, minced
- 1 bell pepper, diced
- 1 teaspoon ground cumin
- 1 teaspoon chili powder
- Salt and pepper to taste
- Corn or flour tortillas
- Toppings: diced avocado, shredded lettuce, salsa, chopped cilantro, lime wedges, etc.

Instructions:

- In a medium saucepan, combine quinoa and water or vegetable broth. Bring to a boil, then reduce heat to low, cover, and simmer for about 15-20 minutes, or until quinoa is cooked and liquid is absorbed. Remove from heat and let it sit covered for 5 minutes, then fluff with a fork.

- While quinoa is cooking, heat olive oil in a large skillet over medium heat. Add diced onion and cook until translucent, about 3-4 minutes. Add minced garlic and cook for another 1-2 minutes, until fragrant.

- Stir in diced bell pepper and cook for about 3-4 minutes, until slightly softened.

- Add the drained and rinsed black beans to the skillet along with the ground cumin, chili powder, salt, and pepper. Cook for another 2-3 minutes, stirring occasionally, until heated through and flavors are combined.

- Once the quinoa is cooked, add it to the skillet with the black bean mixture. Stir to combine and cook for another 2-3 minutes to allow the flavors to meld together. Adjust seasoning if needed.

- Warm the tortillas in a dry skillet or microwave according to package instructions.

- To assemble the tacos, spoon some of the black bean and quinoa mixture onto each tortilla. Top with your desired toppings such as diced avocado, shredded lettuce, salsa, chopped cilantro, and a squeeze of fresh lime juice. Serve immediately and enjoy your nutritious and flavorful Black Bean and Quinoa Tacos!

This recipe provides a balanced combination of protein, fiber, and healthy fats, which can be beneficial for individuals with ADHD and autism. Additionally, the use of whole ingredients and customizable toppings allows for flexibility based on individual preferences and dietary needs.

69. Cauliflower steaks

Cauliflower Steaks with Herbed Quinoa

- Ingredients:
- 1 large head of cauliflower
- 2-3 tablespoons olive oil
- Salt and pepper to taste
- 1 cup quinoa, rinsed
- 2 cups vegetable broth or water
- 2 tablespoons chopped fresh herbs (such as parsley, basil, or thyme)
- 2 cloves garlic, minced
- Juice of 1 lemon
- Optional toppings: chopped nuts, dried cranberries, crumbled feta cheese, etc.

Instructions:

- Preheat your oven to 400°F (200°C).

- Remove the leaves and trim the stem of the cauliflower, leaving the core intact. Carefully slice the cauliflower into 1-inch thick slices to create 'steaks.' You should be able to get 2-3 steaks from one head of cauliflower, depending on its size.

- Place the cauliflower steaks on a baking sheet lined with parchment paper. Brush both sides of the steaks with olive oil and season with salt and pepper to taste.

- Roast the cauliflower steaks in the preheated oven for 20-25 minutes, flipping halfway through, until tender and golden brown.

- While the cauliflower is roasting, prepare the herbed quinoa. In a medium saucepan, combine the rinsed quinoa and vegetable broth or water. Bring to a boil, then reduce heat to low, cover, and simmer for 15-20 minutes, or until quinoa is cooked and liquid is absorbed.

- Once the quinoa is cooked, remove from heat and let it sit covered for 5 minutes. Then, fluff the quinoa with a fork and stir in the chopped fresh herbs, minced garlic, and lemon juice. Season with salt and pepper to taste.

- To serve, place a generous spoonful of herbed quinoa on each plate and top with a cauliflower steak. Garnish with your choice of optional toppings such as chopped nuts, dried cranberries, or crumbled feta cheese. Serve the cauliflower steaks hot and enjoy!

This recipe provides a nutritious and satisfying meal that's rich in fiber, vitamins, and minerals. The cauliflower steaks offer a hearty texture, while the herbed quinoa adds protein and flavor. Plus, you can easily customize the toppings to suit individual preferences and dietary needs.

70. Sweet potato and black bean enchiladas

Ingredients:
- 2 medium sweet potatoes, peeled and diced
- 1 can (15 oz) black beans, drained and rinsed
- 1 bell pepper, diced
- 1 small onion, diced
- 2 cloves garlic, minced
- 1 teaspoon ground cumin
- 1 teaspoon chili powder
- Salt and pepper to taste
- 1 cup enchilada sauce (store-bought or homemade)
- 8-10 small corn tortillas
- 1 cup shredded cheese (such as cheddar or Mexican blend)
- Optional toppings: diced avocado, chopped cilantro, sour cream, salsa, etc.

Instructions:
- Preheat your oven to 375°F (190°C). Lightly grease a 9x13-inch baking dis with cooking spray or olive oil.

- In a large skillet, heat a tablespoon of olive oil over medium heat. Add diced sweet potatoes and cook for about 8-10 minutes, or until tender, stirring occasionally.

- Add diced bell pepper and onion to the skillet with the sweet potatoes. Cook for another 3-4 minutes, until the vegetables are softened.

- Stir in minced garlic, ground cumin, chili powder, salt, and pepper. Cook for another 1-2 minutes, until fragrant.

- Add the drained and rinsed black beans to the skillet and stir to combine with the vegetable mixture. Cook for another 2-3 minutes, until heated through. Remove from heat. Spread a thin layer of enchilada sauce on the bottom of the prepared baking dish.

- Warm the corn tortillas in the microwave for about 30 seconds to make them more pliable. Spoon a portion of the sweet potato and black bean mixture onto each tortilla and roll it up tightly. Place the filled tortillas seam-side down in the baking dish.

- Once all the tortillas are filled and arranged in the baking dish, pour the remaining enchilada sauce evenly over the top. Sprinkle shredded cheese on top of the enchiladas.

- Cover the baking dish with aluminum foil and bake in the preheated oven for 20-25 minutes, or until the enchiladas are heated through and the cheese is melted and bubbly.

- Remove the foil and bake for an additional 5 minutes to lightly brown the cheese. Serve the sweet potato and black bean enchiladas hot, garnished with your choice of toppings such as diced avocado, chopped cilantro, sour cream, or salsa.

71. Zucchini fritters

Ingredients:
- 2 medium zucchinis, grated
- 1 teaspoon salt
- 1 small carrot, grated (optional)
- 1/2 teaspoon black pepper
- 1/2 teaspoon baking powder
- Olive oil for frying
- 1/4 cup finely chopped onion
- 2 cloves garlic, minced
- 1/4 cup chopped fresh herbs (such as parsley, dill, or chives)
- 1/2 cup whole wheat flour or gluten-free flour
- 1/4 cup grated Parmesan cheese (optional)
- 2 large eggs, beaten

Instructions:
- Place the grated zucchini in a colander and sprinkle with salt. Let it sit for about 10 minutes to draw out excess moisture.

- After 10 minutes, use a clean kitchen towel or cheesecloth to squeeze out as much moisture as possible from the grated zucchini. This step is crucial for ensuring the fritters are crispy.

- In a large bowl, combine the grated zucchini, grated carrot (if using), chopped onion, minced garlic, and chopped fresh herbs. Mix well.

- Add the flour, grated Parmesan cheese (if using), beaten eggs, black pepper, and baking powder to the vegetable mixture. Stir until well combined. The batter should be thick but not too dry; if it's too wet, add a bit more flour. Heat a few tablespoons of olive oil in a large skillet over medium heat.

- Scoop about 2 tablespoons of batter for each fritter and drop it into the hot skillet. Use the back of a spoon to flatten the batter into a round fritter shape.

- Cook the fritters for 3-4 minutes on each side, or until they are golden brown and crispy. Adjust the heat as necessary to prevent burning.

- Transfer the cooked fritters to a paper towel-lined plate to drain any excess oil. Repeat with the remaining batter, adding more oil to the skillet as needed. Serve the zucchini fritters warm, with optional toppings or dips such as Greek yogurt, tzatziki sauce, or a squeeze of lemon juice.

These zucchini fritters are a great way to incorporate vegetables into a meal in a way that's both tasty and fun to eat. The use of whole ingredients provides a balanced mix of nutrients, which can be beneficial for individuals with ADHD and autism.

72. Grilled chicken with quinoa

Ingredients:

- 4 boneless, skinless chicken breasts
- 2 tablespoons olive oil
- 2 cloves garlic, minced
- 1 teaspoon paprika
- 1 teaspoon dried oregano
- Salt and pepper to taste
- 1 cup quinoa, rinsed
- 2 cups chicken broth or water
- Juice of 1 lemon
- Chopped fresh parsley for garnish (optional)

Instructions:

- Preheat your grill to medium-high heat. In a small bowl, combine the olive oil, minced garlic, paprika, dried oregano, salt, and pepper to create a marinade for the chicken.

- Place the chicken breasts in a shallow dish and pour the marinade over them, ensuring they are evenly coated. Let the chicken marinate for at least 15-30 minutes, or up to overnight in the refrigerator for maximum flavor.

- While the chicken is marinating, rinse the quinoa under cold water using a fine-mesh sieve. This helps remove any bitter coating.

- In a medium saucepan, bring the chicken broth or water to a boil. Stir in the rinsed quinoa and reduce the heat to low. Cover and simmer for about 15-20 minutes, or until the quinoa is cooked and the liquid is absorbed. Fluff the quinoa with a fork and remove it from the heat.

- Once the grill is preheated, grill the marinated chicken breasts for about 6-8 minutes per side, or until they are cooked through and no longer pink in the center. Cooking time may vary depending on the thickness of the chicken breasts. Remove the grilled chicken from the grill and let it rest for a few minutes before slicing.

- To serve, spoon a portion of cooked quinoa onto each plate and top with sliced grilled chicken breasts. Drizzle with fresh lemon juice and garnish with chopped fresh parsley, if desired. Serve the grilled chicken with quinoa immediately, and enjoy!

This recipe provides a good balance of protein, carbohydrates, and healthy fats, making it a nutritious and well-rounded meal option. The grilled chicken is flavorful and juicy, while the quinoa adds a satisfying texture and serves as a nutritious base. Plus, the simple preparation makes it easy to customize with your favorite herbs and spices.

74. Almond flour pancakes

Ingredients:
- 1 1/2 cups almond flour
- 1/2 teaspoon baking soda
- 1/4 teaspoon salt
- 3 large eggs
- 1/4 cup unsweetened almond milk (or any milk of choice)
- 1 tablespoon maple syrup or honey (optional)
- 1 teaspoon vanilla extract
- Coconut oil or butter for cooking

Instructions:

- In a medium bowl, whisk together the almond flour, baking soda, and salt.

- In a separate bowl, whisk the eggs, almond milk, maple syrup (if using), and vanilla extract until well combined.

- Pour the wet ingredients into the dry ingredients and stir until just combined. Let the batter sit for a few minutes to thicken.

- Heat a non-stick skillet or griddle over medium heat and add a little coconut oil or butter.

- Scoop about 1/4 cup of batter onto the skillet for each pancake. Spread the batter slightly with the back of a spoon to form a round shape.

- Cook the pancakes for 2-3 minutes on each side, or until bubbles form on the surface and the edges are set. Flip and cook for an additional 2-3 minutes, until golden brown and cooked through.

- Transfer the cooked pancakes to a plate and keep warm. Repeat with the remaining batter, adding more oil or butter as needed.

- Serve the almond flour pancakes warm with your favorite toppings such as fresh berries, sliced bananas, a drizzle of maple syrup, or a dollop of yogurt.

These almond flour pancakes are a great alternative to traditional pancakes, offering a good source of protein and healthy fats, which can help with sustained energy levels and focus. Plus, they're easy to make and delicious!

75. Gluten-free pizza with vegetable toppings

Ingredients:
- 1 gluten-free pizza crust
(store-bought or homemade)
- 1/2 cup tomato sauce or pizza sauce
- 1 cup shredded mozzarella cheese
(or dairy-free alternative)

Instructions:
- Preheat your oven according to the
instructions for the gluten-free pizza crust.

- Assorted vegetable toppings (such as sliced bell peppers, mushrooms, red onions, spinach, cherry tomatoes, olives, etc.)
- Olive oil
- Salt and pepper to taste
- Optional toppings: fresh basil, crushed red pepper flakes, grated Parmesan cheese (if tolerated), etc.

- If using a homemade gluten-free pizza crust, prepare the crust according to the recipe instructions. If using a store-bought crust, follow the package instructions for pre-baking, if necessary.

- Once the crust is ready, spread a layer of tomato sauce or pizza sauce evenly over the surface, leaving a small border around the edges. Sprinkle shredded mozzarella cheese evenly over the sauce.

- Arrange your desired vegetable toppings over the cheese, distributing them evenly across the pizza. Drizzle a little olive oil over the vegetable toppings and season with salt and pepper to taste.

- If using a pre-baked crust, place the assembled pizza directly on a baking sheet or pizza stone. If using a raw crust, follow the package instructions for baking.

- Bake the pizza in the preheated oven according to the crust instructions, or until the cheese is melted and bubbly, and the crust is golden brown.

- Once the pizza is cooked, remove it from the oven and let it cool for a few minutes before slicing. Garnish the pizza with optional toppings such as fresh basil, crushed red pepper flakes, or grated Parmesan cheese, if desired. Slice the pizza into wedges and serve warm.

This gluten-free pizza with vegetable toppings offers a flavorful and nutritious meal option that's packed with vitamins, minerals, and fiber from the vegetables. Plus, the use of a gluten-free crust ensures that it's suitable for individuals with gluten sensitivities or celiac disease. Feel free to customize the toppings based on personal preferences and dietary needs!

76. Grilled portobello mushrooms

Ingredients:
- 4 large portobello mushrooms
- 1/4 cup olive oil
- 2 tablespoons balsamic vinegar
- 2 cloves garlic, minced
- 1 teaspoon dried oregano
- Salt and pepper to taste
- Fresh parsley or basil for garnish (optional)

Instructions:
- Clean the portobello mushrooms by wiping them with a damp paper towel. Remove the stems and gently scrape out the gills with a spoon.

- In a small bowl, whisk together the olive oil, balsamic vinegar, minced garlic, dried oregano, salt, and pepper to create the marinade.

- Place the mushrooms in a shallow dish or a resealable plastic bag and pour the marinade over them. Ensure that each mushroom is evenly coated. Let the mushrooms marinate for at least 15-30 minutes, or up to 2 hours for more flavor. Preheat your grill to medium-high heat.

- Once the grill is hot, place the marinated mushrooms cap-side down on the grill. Cook for about 5-7 minutes on each side, or until they are tender and have nice grill marks. Baste the mushrooms with any remaining marinade during grilling.

- Remove the mushrooms from the grill and let them rest for a few minutes. Garnish with fresh parsley or basil if desired, and serve warm.

Serving Suggestions:
- As a Main Dish: Serve the grilled portobello mushrooms with a side of quinoa, brown rice, or a fresh salad for a complete meal.

- As a Sandwich: Place the grilled mushrooms on a gluten-free bun with your favorite toppings, such as lettuce, tomato, avocado, and a spread of your choice.

- As a Side Dish: Serve alongside grilled chicken, fish, or a veggie platter for a delicious accompaniment.

Grilled portobello mushrooms are a versatile and nutrient-rich option that can be easily incorporated into various meals. The marinade adds a burst of flavor while keeping the dish simple and healthy. This recipe is also great for those following gluten-free, vegetarian, or vegan diets.

77. Shrimp and avocado salad

Ingredients:
- 1 lb large shrimp, peeled and deveined
- 1 tablespoon olive oil
- Salt and pepper to taste
- 1 teaspoon garlic powder
- 2 ripe avocados, diced
- 1 cup cherry tomatoes, halved
- 1 small red onion, finely diced
- 1 cucumber, diced
- 1/4 cup fresh cilantro, chopped
- Juice of 2 limes
- 2 tablespoons extra virgin olive oil
- 1 teaspoon honey or agave syrup (optional)
- 1/2 teaspoon ground cumin
- Mixed greens or lettuce (optional)

Instructions:

Cook the Shrimp:
- In a bowl, toss the shrimp with 1 tablespoon of olive oil, garlic powder, salt, and pepper.

- Heat a skillet over medium-high heat. Add the shrimp and cook for 2-3 minutes on each side, or until they are pink and opaque. Remove from heat and let them cool.

Prepare the Salad: In a large salad bowl, combine the diced avocados, cherry tomatoes, red onion, cucumber, and chopped cilantro. Add the cooled shrimp to the salad bowl.

Make the Dressing: In a small bowl, whisk together the lime juice, extra virgin olive oil, honey (if using), ground cumin, salt, and pepper to taste.

Assemble the Salad: Pour the dressing over the shrimp and vegetable mixture. Toss gently to combine all the ingredients and coat them with the dressing.

If desired, serve the shrimp and avocado salad over a bed of mixed greens or lettuce for added texture and nutrition.

Garnish with extra cilantro or a squeeze of lime juice if desired.

This shrimp and avocado salad is light, refreshing, and packed with healthy fats, protein, and a variety of vitamins and minerals. The combination of shrimp and avocado provides a satisfying texture and flavor, while the fresh vegetables and lime dressing add brightness and acidity. It's a perfect meal for a balanced diet and can be enjoyed as a lunch or dinner option.

78. Rice paper spring rolls

Ingredients:
- Rice paper wrappers (available at Asian grocery stores or online)
- Cooked vermicelli rice noodles (optional)
- Assorted fillings:
- Thinly sliced vegetables (such as carrots, cucumbers, bell peppers, lettuce, and avocado)
- Fresh herbs (such as cilantro, mint, and basil)
- Cooked protein (such as shrimp, chicken, tofu, or tempeh)
- Optional extras (such as sliced mango, avocado, or crunchy toppings like peanuts or sesame seeds)
- Warm water for soaking rice paper wrappers
- Dipping sauce of your choice (such as peanut sauce, sweet chili sauce, hoisin sauce, or soy sauce)

Instructions:
Prepare the Fillings: Prepare all the fillings by washing, slicing, and chopping them into thin strips or bite-sized pieces. Cook any protein if using.

Soak the Rice Paper Wrappers:
- Fill a shallow dish or pie plate with warm water.

- Dip one rice paper wrapper into the warm water for about 5-10 seconds, or until it becomes soft and pliable. Be careful not to soak it for too long, as it will become too fragile to work with.

Assemble the Spring Rolls:
- Place the softened rice paper wrapper on a clean, damp kitchen towel or a smooth surface.

- Arrange a small amount of each filling in the center of the wrapper, leaving some space on the sides.

- Fold the sides of the wrapper over the filling, then fold the bottom edge over the filling tightly, and continue rolling until you reach the top edge. Roll it tightly to ensure that the filling is secure. Repeat the process with the remaining rice paper wrappers and fillings.

Serve the rice paper spring rolls immediately with dipping sauce of your choice.

Tips:
- Work with one rice paper wrapper at a time to prevent them from sticking together. Keep the fillings well-distributed and not too bulky to make rolling easier. Experiment with different combinations of fillings and dipping sauces to suit your taste preferences.

79. Gluten-free meatballs

Ingredients:

- 1 lb ground meat (beef, turkey, chicken, or pork)
- 1/2 cup gluten-free breadcrumbs or rolled oats (certified gluten-free)
- 1/4 cup grated Parmesan cheese (optional)
- 1/4 cup finely chopped fresh parsley
- 1/4 cup finely chopped onion
- 2 cloves garlic, minced
- 1 large egg
- 1 teaspoon dried oregano
- 1 teaspoon dried basil
- Salt and pepper to taste
- Olive oil for cooking

Instructions:

- Preheat your oven to 375°F (190°C).

- In a large mixing bowl, combine the ground meat, gluten-free breadcrumbs or rolled oats, grated Parmesan cheese (if using), chopped parsley, chopped onion, minced garlic, egg, dried oregano, dried basil, salt, and pepper. Use your hands to mix until all ingredients are well combined.

- Shape the meat mixture into golf ball-sized meatballs, rolling them between your palms. Place the meatballs on a baking sheet lined with parchment paper or aluminum foil, spacing them evenly apart.

- Drizzle the meatballs with a little olive oil to help them brown and crisp up in the oven.

- Bake the meatballs in the preheated oven for 20-25 minutes, or until they are cooked through and lightly browned on the outside. The internal temperature should reach 160°F (71°C) for ground beef and pork, and 165°F (74°C) for ground turkey and chicken.

- Once the meatballs are cooked, remove them from the oven and let them rest for a few minutes before serving.

- Serve the gluten-free meatballs with your favorite sauce, such as marinara sauce, barbecue sauce, or gravy. They can be enjoyed on their own as a snack, appetizer, or as part of a main meal with pasta, rice, or vegetables.

These gluten-free meatballs are packed with flavor and protein, making them a satisfying and nutritious option for individuals with ADHD and autism. Plus, they're easy to make and can be customized with different herbs, spices, and sauces to suit your taste preferences.

80. Coconut flour banana bread

Ingredients:
4 ripe bananas, mashed
4 large eggs
1/4 cup coconut oil, melted
1/4 cup honey or maple syrup
1 teaspoon vanilla extract
1/2 cup coconut flour
1 teaspoon baking powder
1/2 teaspoon baking soda
1/2 teaspoon ground cinnamon
1/4 teaspoon salt
Optional add-ins: chopped nuts, chocolate chips, shredded coconut, etc.

Instructions:
- Preheat your oven to 350°F (175°C). Grease or line a 9x5-inch loaf pan with parchment paper. In a large mixing bowl, mash the ripe bananas with a fork until smooth.

- Add the eggs, melted coconut oil, honey or maple syrup, and vanilla extract to the mashed bananas. Mix well until all ingredients are combined. In a separate bowl, whisk together the coconut flour, baking powder, baking soda, ground cinnamon, and salt.

- Gradually add the dry ingredients to the wet ingredients, stirring until a smooth batter forms. Be careful not to overmix. If using any optional add-ins such as chopped nuts or chocolate chips, fold them into the batter.

- Pour the batter into the prepared loaf pan and spread it evenly with a spatula.

- Bake in the preheated oven for 45-55 minutes, or until the top is golden brown and a toothpick inserted into the center comes out clean.

- Remove the banana bread from the oven and let it cool in the pan for about 10 minutes. Then, transfer it to a wire rack to cool completely before slicing.

- Once cooled, slice the coconut flour banana bread and serve. Enjoy it as a snack, breakfast, or dessert!

This coconut flour banana bread is moist, flavorful, and perfect for individuals with ADHD and autism. It's made with wholesome ingredients and can be easily customized with your favorite add-ins. Plus, it's a great way to use up ripe bananas and satisfy your sweet cravings in a healthier way.

81. Almond milk smoothie

Ingredients:
- 1 cup unsweetened almond milk
- 1 ripe banana, frozen
- 1/2 cup frozen berries (such as strawberries, blueberries, raspberries, or a mix)
- 1 tablespoon almond butter or peanut butter (optional)
- 1 tablespoon chia seeds or flaxseeds (optional)
- 1 tablespoon honey or maple syrup (optional, for sweetness)
- Ice cubes (optional, for a colder smoothie)

Instructions:

- In a blender, combine the unsweetened almond milk, frozen banana, frozen berries, almond butter or peanut butter (if using), chia seeds or flaxseeds (if using), and honey or maple syrup (if using).

- If desired, add a handful of ice cubes to the blender for a colder smoothie.

- Blend all the ingredients together until smooth and creamy. If the smoothie is too thick, you can add more almond milk or a splash of water to reach your desired consistency.

- Taste the smoothie and adjust the sweetness if needed by adding more honey or maple syrup.

- Once the smoothie is well blended and the desired consistency is reached, pour it into glasses and serve immediately.

- Optionally, garnish the smoothie with additional toppings such as sliced fruit, chopped nuts, or a sprinkle of cinnamon.

This almond milk smoothie is a nutritious and satisfying option for individuals with ADHD and autism. It's rich in vitamins, minerals, and antioxidants from the fruit and seeds, and the almond milk provides a creamy texture without dairy. Plus, it's easy to customize with your favorite ingredients and can be enjoyed as a quick breakfast, snack, or post-workout refuel.

82. Coconut yogurt with berries

Ingredients:
- 1 cup unsweetened coconut yogurt (store-bought or homemade)
- Assorted fresh berries (such as strawberries, blueberries, raspberries, blackberries)
- Optional toppings: sliced bananas, chopped nuts, shredded coconut, honey or maple syrup for drizzling

Instructions:
- If using store-bought coconut yogurt, give it a good stir to ensure it's well mixed and creamy. If making homemade coconut yogurt, prepare it according to your preferred recipe and allow it to chill in the refrigerator until ready to use.

- Wash and prepare the fresh berries by rinsing them under cold water and patting them dry with a paper towel. You can slice larger berries like strawberries if desired.

- In serving bowls or glasses, spoon a portion of the coconut yogurt.

- Arrange the fresh berries on top of the coconut yogurt.

- If desired, add any optional toppings such as sliced bananas, chopped nuts, shredded coconut, or a drizzle of honey or maple syrup for sweetness.

- Serve the coconut yogurt with berries immediately and enjoy!

This coconut yogurt with berries is a refreshing and nutritious option for individuals with ADHD and autism. Coconut yogurt is dairy-free and rich in probiotics, which can support gut health and digestion. Fresh berries provide vitamins, minerals, and antioxidants, making this dish a great choice for a balanced and satisfying snack or breakfast. Plus, it's easy to customize with your favorite toppings and can be enjoyed any time of the day.

83. Dairy-free mac and cheese

Ingredients:

- 8 oz (about 2 cups) elbow macaroni or any pasta of your choice (gluten-free if needed)
- 1 cup raw cashews, soaked in water for at least 4 hours or overnight
- 1 cup unsweetened almond milk or other non-dairy milk
- 1/4 cup nutritional yeast
- 2 tablespoons lemon juice
- 2 cloves garlic, minced
- 1 teaspoon Dijon mustard
- 1/2 teaspoon onion powder
- 1/2 teaspoon paprika
- Salt and pepper to taste
- Optional add-ins: steamed broccoli, diced tomatoes, cooked peas, sautéed mushrooms, etc.

Instructions:

- Cook the pasta according to the package instructions until al dente. Drain and set aside.

- In a blender, combine the soaked cashews, almond milk, nutritional yeast, lemon juice, minced garlic, Dijon mustard, onion powder, paprika, salt, and pepper.

- Blend the ingredients until smooth and creamy, scraping down the sides of the blender as needed. If the sauce is too thick, you can add more almond milk to reach your desired consistency.

- Taste the sauce and adjust the seasonings if needed, adding more salt, pepper, or lemon juice to taste.

- In a large mixing bowl, toss the cooked pasta with the dairy-free cheese sauce until evenly coated.

- If desired, add any optional add-ins such as steamed broccoli, diced tomatoes, cooked peas, sautéed mushrooms, etc., and gently mix to combine.

- Serve the dairy-free mac and cheese immediately, garnished with chopped parsley or extra nutritional yeast if desired.

This dairy-free mac and cheese is creamy, flavorful, and satisfying, making it a great comfort food option for individuals with ADHD and autism. The cashew-based cheese sauce provides a creamy texture and cheesy flavor without the need for dairy. Plus, it's easy to customize with your favorite add-ins to make it even more delicious and nutritious.

84. Grilled tofu with vegetables

Ingredients:
- 1 block (14-16 oz) extra-firm tofu, pressed and drained
- 2 tablespoons soy sauce or tamari (gluten-free if needed)
- 2 tablespoons olive oil
- 1 tablespoon maple syrup or honey
- 2 cloves garlic, minced
- 1 teaspoon grated ginger
- 1/2 teaspoon ground cumin
- 1/2 teaspoon smoked paprika
- Salt and pepper to taste
- Assorted vegetables for grilling (such as bell peppers, zucchini, mushrooms, onions, cherry tomatoes)
- Olive oil for brushing

Instructions:
- Preheat your grill to medium-high heat.

- While the grill is heating, prepare the tofu. Cut the pressed tofu into slices or cubes, depending on your preference.

- In a small bowl, whisk together the soy sauce or tamari, olive oil, maple syrup or honey, minced garlic, grated ginger, ground cumin, smoked paprika, salt, and pepper to make the marinade.

- Place the tofu pieces in a shallow dish or a resealable plastic bag, and pour the marinade over them. Ensure that the tofu is evenly coated with the marinade. Let it marinate for at least 15-30 minutes, or longer if time allows.

- While the tofu is marinating, prepare the vegetables for grilling. Wash and chop the vegetables into bite-sized pieces, ensuring they are all roughly the same size for even cooking.

- Thread the marinated tofu pieces and chopped vegetables onto skewers, alternating between tofu and vegetables.

- Brush the grill grates with a little olive oil to prevent sticking. Place the tofu and vegetable skewers on the grill.

- Grill the tofu and vegetables for 4-5 minutes on each side, or until they are lightly charred and tender, basting with any remaining marinade while grilling.

- Once the tofu and vegetables are grilled to your liking, remove them from the grill and transfer them to a serving platter. Serve the grilled tofu and vegetables hot, garnished with chopped fresh herbs if desired.

85. Coconut curry chicken

Ingredients:
- 1 lb boneless, skinless chicken breasts or thighs, cut into bite-sized pieces
- 1 tablespoon coconut oil or olive oil
- 1 onion, diced
- 2 cloves garlic, minced
- 1 tablespoon grated ginger
- 2 tablespoons curry powder
- 1 teaspoon ground turmeric
- 1 teaspoon ground cumin
- 1 teaspoon ground coriander
- 1 can (13.5 oz) coconut milk
- 1 cup chicken broth
- 2 cups mixed vegetables (such as bell peppers, carrots, peas, and potatoes)
- Salt and pepper to taste
- Fresh cilantro for garnish (optional)
- Cooked rice or naan bread for serving

Instructions:
- Heat the coconut oil or olive oil in a large skillet or Dutch oven over medium heat. Add the diced onion to the skillet and sauté until softened, about 3-4 minutes.

- Stir in the minced garlic and grated ginger, and cook for another 1-2 minutes until fragrant.

- Add the curry powder, ground turmeric, ground cumin, and ground coriander to the skillet. Cook, stirring constantly, for about 1 minute to toast the spices.

- Add the chicken pieces to the skillet and cook until they are lightly browned on all sides, about 5-6 minutes.

- Pour in the coconut milk and chicken broth, stirring to combine. Bring the mixture to a simmer.

- Add the mixed vegetables to the skillet and stir to combine. Reduce the heat to low, cover, and simmer for about 15-20 minutes, or until the chicken is cooked through and the vegetables are tender.

- Season the coconut curry chicken with salt and pepper to taste. Serve the coconut curry chicken hot, garnished with fresh cilantro if desired, and accompanied by cooked rice or naan bread.

This coconut curry chicken is creamy, aromatic, and packed with flavor from the combination of spices and coconut milk. It's a satisfying and nutritious meal option for individuals with ADHD and autism, providing a good balance of protein, healthy fats, and vegetables. Plus, it's easy to customize with your favorite vegetables and spice levels to suit your taste preferences. Enjoy this comforting dish for a delicious and comforting meal!

86. Avocado chocolate mousse

Ingredients:
- 2 ripe avocados, peeled and pitted
- 1/4 cup unsweetened cocoa powder
- 1/4 cup maple syrup or honey
- 1 teaspoon vanilla extract
- Pinch of salt
- Optional toppings: sliced strawberries, raspberries, shaved chocolate, chopped nuts, or whipped coconut cream

Instructions:

- In a food processor or blender, combine the ripe avocados, unsweetened cocoa powder, maple syrup or honey, vanilla extract, and a pinch of salt.

- Blend the ingredients until smooth and creamy, scraping down the sides of the bowl as needed to ensure everything is well combined.

- Taste the chocolate mousse and adjust the sweetness if needed by adding more maple syrup or honey.

- Once the avocado chocolate mousse is smooth and sweetened to your liking, transfer it to serving bowls or glasses.

- Cover the bowls or glasses with plastic wrap and refrigerate the avocado chocolate mousse for at least 30 minutes to chill and firm up.

- When ready to serve, remove the avocado chocolate mousse from the refrigerator and garnish with your favorite toppings such as sliced strawberries, raspberries, shaved chocolate, chopped nuts, or whipped coconut cream.

- Serve the avocado chocolate mousse immediately and enjoy!

This avocado chocolate mousse is rich, creamy, and decadent, with a luscious texture that's reminiscent of traditional chocolate mousse. It's naturally sweetened with maple syrup or honey and packed with healthy fats from the avocados, making it a satisfying and nutritious dessert option for individuals with ADHD and autism. Plus, it's easy to customize with your favorite toppings to add extra flavor and texture. Enjoy this delicious treat as a guilt-free indulgence!

87. Dairy-free cheese quesadillas

Ingredients:
- 4 large flour tortillas (gluten-free if needed)
- 1 cup dairy-free cheese shreds (such as Daiya, Violife, or Follow Your Heart)
- 1/2 cup cooked black beans (optional)
- 1/2 cup corn kernels (fresh, frozen, or canned)
- 1/4 cup diced bell peppers
- 1/4 cup diced red onion
- 1 teaspoon ground cumin
- 1/2 teaspoon chili powder
- Salt and pepper to taste
- Olive oil or dairy-free butter for cooking
- Salsa, guacamole, dairy-free sour cream, or chopped cilantro for serving (optional)

Instructions:
- In a large mixing bowl, combine the cooked black beans (if using), corn kernels, diced bell peppers, diced red onion, ground cumin, chili powder, salt, and pepper. Stir until well combined.

- Heat a large skillet or griddle over medium heat. Lightly brush one side of a flour tortilla with olive oil or spread dairy-free butter on it.

- Place the tortilla, oil/butter side down, in the skillet or griddle. Sprinkle a quarter of the dairy-free cheese shreds evenly over the tortilla.

- Spoon a quarter of the vegetable and bean mixture over half of the tortilla. Fold the tortilla in half to cover the filling, creating a half-moon shape.

- Cook the quesadilla for 2-3 minutes on each side, or until golden brown and crispy, and the cheese is melted. Repeat the process with the remaining tortillas and filling ingredients. Once all the quesadillas are cooked, transfer them to a cutting board and slice each one into wedges.

- Serve the dairy-free cheese quesadillas hot, with salsa, guacamole, dairy-free sour cream, or chopped cilantro for dipping or garnish, if desired.

These dairy-free cheese quesadillas are deliciously cheesy, flavorful, and customizable with your favorite fillings. They are perfect for a quick and easy lunch, dinner, or snack option that's suitable for individuals with ADHD and autism who need to avoid dairy. Plus, they can be made ahead of time and stored in the refrigerator for a convenient meal option. Enjoy these tasty quesadillas as a satisfying and nutritious meal!

88. Cashew cream sauce pasta

Ingredients:
- 8 oz (about 225g) pasta of your choice (such as spaghetti, fettuccine, penne, or gluten-free pasta)
- 1 cup raw cashews, soaked in water for at least 4 hours or overnight
- 1 cup vegetable broth or water
- 2 cloves garlic, minced
- 2 tablespoons nutritional yeast (optional, for a cheesy flavor)
- 1 tablespoon lemon juice
- Salt and pepper to taste
- Optional add-ins: sautéed vegetables, cooked protein (such as chicken, shrimp, or tofu), fresh herbs, cherry tomatoes, etc.

Instructions:
- Cook the pasta according to the package instructions until al dente. Drain and set aside.

- While the pasta is cooking, drain the soaked cashews and rinse them under cold water.

- In a blender or food processor, combine the soaked cashews, vegetable broth or water, minced garlic, nutritional yeast (if using), lemon juice, salt, and pepper.

- Blend the ingredients until smooth and creamy, scraping down the sides of the blender or food processor as needed to ensure everything is well combined. If the sauce is too thick, you can add more vegetable broth or water to reach your desired consistency.

- Taste the cashew cream sauce and adjust the seasoning if needed, adding more salt, pepper, or lemon juice to taste.

- Once the pasta is cooked and drained, return it to the pot or transfer it to a large serving bowl. Pour the cashew cream sauce over the cooked pasta and toss to coat evenly.

- If desired, add any optional add-ins such as sautéed vegetables, cooked protein, fresh herbs, cherry tomatoes, etc., and gently mix to combine. Serve the cashew cream sauce pasta hot, garnished with additional fresh herbs or nutritional yeast if desired.

This cashew cream sauce pasta is rich, creamy, and packed with flavor, making it a satisfying and nutritious meal option for individuals with ADHD and autism. The creamy cashew sauce provides a dairy-free alternative to traditional cream-based sauces, and it pairs perfectly with pasta and your favorite add-ins. Plus, it's easy to customize with different vegetables, proteins, and herbs to suit your taste preferences. Enjoy this delicious and comforting dish for a satisfying meal!

89. Roasted chickpeas

Ingredients:

- 1 can (15 oz) chickpeas (also known as garbanzo beans), drained and rinsed
- 1 tablespoon olive oil or melted coconut oil
- 1 teaspoon ground cumin
- 1 teaspoon paprika
- 1/2 teaspoon garlic powder
- 1/2 teaspoon onion powder
- 1/4 teaspoon cayenne pepper (optional, for a spicy kick)
- Salt to taste

Instructions:

- Preheat your oven to 400°F (200°C). Line a baking sheet with parchment paper or aluminum foil for easy cleanup.

- Drain and rinse the chickpeas under cold water. Pat them dry with a clean kitchen towel or paper towels to remove excess moisture.

- In a mixing bowl, toss the dried chickpeas with olive oil or melted coconut oil until they are evenly coated.

- In a small bowl, combine the ground cumin, paprika, garlic powder, onion powder, cayenne pepper (if using), and salt.

- Sprinkle the spice mixture over the oiled chickpeas, tossing to coat them evenly.

- Spread the seasoned chickpeas out in a single layer on the prepared baking sheet.

- Roast the chickpeas in the preheated oven for 25-30 minutes, or until they are crispy and golden brown, shaking the pan halfway through baking to ensure even cooking.

- Once the chickpeas are roasted to your desired level of crispiness, remove them from the oven and let them cool on the baking sheet for a few minutes.

- Serve the roasted chickpeas warm as a snack, or let them cool completely before storing them in an airtight container for later enjoyment.

These roasted chickpeas are crunchy, savory, and packed with flavor from the spices. They make a delicious and satisfying snack for individuals with ADHD and autism, providing a good source of protein, fiber, and nutrients. Plus, they're easy to customize with your favorite spices and seasonings to suit your taste preferences. Enjoy these roasted chickpeas as a healthy and satisfying snack option!

90. Almond milk chia pudding

Ingredients:
- 1/4 cup chia seeds
- 1 cup unsweetened almond milk (or any other non-dairy milk of your choice)
- 1 tablespoon maple syrup or honey (optional, for sweetness)
- 1/2 teaspoon vanilla extract
- Optional toppings: fresh berries, sliced fruits, nuts, seeds, shredded coconut, or a drizzle of honey or maple syrup

Instructions:
- In a mixing bowl or glass jar, combine the chia seeds, unsweetened almond milk, maple syrup or honey (if using), and vanilla extract.

- Stir the mixture well to ensure the chia seeds are evenly distributed and not clumped together.

- Cover the bowl or jar and refrigerate the chia seed mixture for at least 2-3 hours, or preferably overnight. During this time, the chia seeds will absorb the liquid and swell, resulting in a thick and creamy pudding-like consistency.

- After the chia pudding has chilled and thickened, give it a good stir to break up any clumps and ensure a smooth texture.

- Serve the almond milk chia pudding in individual bowls or glasses, and top with your favorite toppings such as fresh berries, sliced fruits, nuts, seeds, shredded coconut, or a drizzle of honey or maple syrup.

- Enjoy the almond milk chia pudding immediately, or store any leftovers in the refrigerator for up to 3-4 days.

This almond milk chia pudding is creamy, satisfying, and packed with fiber, protein, and healthy fats from the chia seeds and almond milk. It's naturally sweetened with maple syrup or honey and can be customized with your favorite toppings to add extra flavor and texture. Plus, it's easy to prepare ahead of time and makes a convenient and nutritious breakfast, snack, or dessert option for individuals with ADHD and autism. Enjoy this delicious and nourishing treat!

91. Veggie sticks with guacamole

Ingredients:

- Assorted vegetables for dipping (such as carrot sticks, cucumber slices, bell pepper strips, celery sticks, cherry tomatoes, snap peas, or radish slices)
- 2 ripe avocados, peeled and pitted
- 1 small ripe tomato, diced
- 1/4 cup diced red onion
- 1 clove garlic, minced
- 1 tablespoon lime juice
- 1/4 teaspoon ground cumin
- Salt and pepper to taste
- Optional add-ins: chopped cilantro, diced jalapeño, diced bell pepper, or a sprinkle of chili powder

Instructions:

- Wash and prepare the assorted vegetables for dipping by slicing them into sticks, slices, or bite-sized pieces.

- In a mixing bowl, mash the ripe avocados with a fork until smooth and creamy.

- Add the diced tomato, diced red onion, minced garlic, lime juice, ground cumin, salt, and pepper to the mashed avocados.

- If desired, add any optional add-ins such as chopped cilantro, diced jalapeño, diced bell pepper, or a sprinkle of chili powder.

- Stir the guacamole mixture until all ingredients are well combined and the desired consistency is reached. Taste and adjust the seasoning if needed by adding more lime juice, salt, or pepper.

- Transfer the guacamole to a serving bowl and garnish with additional chopped cilantro or a sprinkle of chili powder if desired.

- Arrange the assorted vegetable sticks on a serving platter or tray alongside the guacamole. Serve the veggie sticks with guacamole immediately and enjoy!

This veggie sticks with guacamole snack is packed with vitamins, minerals, and healthy fats from the vegetables and avocado. It's a satisfying and nutritious option for individuals with ADHD and autism, providing a good balance of flavors and textures. Plus, it's easy to customize with your favorite vegetables and add-ins to suit your taste preferences. Enjoy this delicious and wholesome snack anytime!

92. Boiled eggs

Ingredients:

Eggs (as many as desired)

Instructions:

- Place the eggs in a single layer in a saucepan or pot. Make sure the eggs are not stacked on top of each other.

- Add enough cold water to the pot to cover the eggs by about 1 inch (2.5 cm). Place the pot on the stove over medium-high heat and bring the water to a rolling boil.

- Once the water is boiling, remove the pot from the heat and cover it with a lid. Let the eggs sit in the hot water for the desired amount of time based on your preference for egg doneness:

- For soft-boiled eggs with a runny yolk: Let the eggs sit in the hot water for 4-6 minutes.

- For medium-boiled eggs with a slightly firm yolk: Let the eggs sit in the hot water for 7-9 minutes.

- For hard-boiled eggs with a fully set yolk: Let the eggs sit in the hot water for 10-12 minutes. While the eggs are sitting in the hot water, prepare a bowl of ice water.

- After the desired cooking time has elapsed, carefully remove the eggs from the hot water using a slotted spoon and transfer them to the bowl of ice water.

- Let the eggs cool in the ice water for a few minutes to stop the cooking process and make them easier to handle.

- Once the eggs are cool enough to handle, gently tap them on a hard surface to crack the shell, then peel away the shell under cold running water.

- Rinse the peeled eggs under cold water to remove any remaining bits of shell. Pat the boiled eggs dry with a clean kitchen towel and serve them whole, sliced, or chopped as desired.

Boiled eggs are a convenient and portable snack that's rich in protein, vitamins, and minerals. They can be enjoyed on their own as a quick and nutritious snack, or added to salads, sandwiches, or other dishes for added flavor and protein. Plus, they can be prepared ahead of time and stored in the refrigerator for easy snacking throughout the week. Enjoy these boiled eggs as a tasty and satisfying snack option!

93. Nuts and seeds

Nuts:
- Almonds
- Walnuts
- Cashews
- Pecans
- Brazil nuts
- Hazelnuts
- Macadamia nuts
- Pistachios

Seeds:
- Pumpkin seeds (pepitas)
- Sunflower seeds
- Chia seeds
- Flaxseeds (ground or whole)
- Hemp seeds
- Sesame seeds
- Poppy seeds

Ways to Enjoy:

- Raw: Enjoy nuts and seeds as they are for a quick and convenient snack.

- Roasted: Roast nuts and seeds with a little bit of salt or your favorite spices for added flavor and crunch.

- Trail Mix: Combine nuts and seeds with dried fruits, coconut flakes, and dark chocolate chips for a tasty trail mix.

- Nut Butter: Spread nut butter (such as almond butter or peanut butter) on whole grain crackers, apple slices, or celery sticks for a satisfying snack.

- Seeds on Salads: Sprinkle seeds on top of salads for added texture and nutrition.

- Smoothies: Blend seeds (such as chia seeds or flaxseeds) into smoothies for an extra boost of fiber and omega-3 fatty acids.

- Homemade Energy Bars: Make homemade energy bars or protein bars using nuts, seeds, dried fruits, and oats for a nutritious snack on the go.

Nuts and seeds are rich in protein, healthy fats, fiber, vitamins, and minerals, making them an excellent choice for supporting overall health and well-being. They can help provide sustained energy, improve focus and concentration, and regulate mood, making them particularly beneficial for individuals with ADHD and autism. However, be mindful of any allergies or sensitivities to nuts and seeds when incorporating them into your diet. Enjoy a variety of nuts and seeds as part of a balanced diet for optimal nutrition and enjoyment!

94. Greek yogurt with a splash of vanilla extract

Ingredients:
Plain Greek yogurt
Vanilla extract

Instructions:

- Spoon the desired amount of plain Greek yogurt into a bowl or serving dish.

- Add a splash of vanilla extract to the Greek yogurt. Start with a small amount and adjust to taste, depending on how strong you want the vanilla flavor to be.

- Stir the Greek yogurt and vanilla extract together until well combined.

- Taste the yogurt and add more vanilla extract if desired, adjusting to your preference for sweetness and flavor.

- Serve the Greek yogurt with a splash of vanilla extract immediately, or cover and refrigerate it for later enjoyment.

Optional Add-Ins:

- Sweeteners: If you prefer a sweeter yogurt, you can add a drizzle of honey, maple syrup, or agave syrup.

- Fresh Fruit: Top the yogurt with sliced fruits such as berries, bananas, peaches, or mangoes for added sweetness and flavor.

- Nuts and Seeds: Sprinkle chopped nuts, seeds, or granola on top of the yogurt for added crunch and texture.

- Cinnamon: Stir in a pinch of ground cinnamon for a warm and comforting flavor.

- Coconut Flakes: Garnish the yogurt with shredded coconut for a tropical twist.

Greek yogurt is a rich source of protein, calcium, and probiotics, making it a nutritious snack option for individuals with ADHD and autism. The addition of vanilla extract provides a delicious and aromatic flavor without the need for added sugars or artificial sweeteners. Plus, this snack is quick and easy to prepare, making it perfect for busy days or as a satisfying treat any time of the day. Enjoy this creamy and flavorful Greek yogurt with a splash of vanilla extract for a tasty and nutritious snack!

95. Cucumber and tomato salad

Ingredients:

- 2 large cucumbers, diced
- 2 large tomatoes, diced
- 1/2 red onion, thinly sliced
- 1/4 cup chopped fresh parsley or cilantro
- 2 tablespoons extra virgin olive oil
- 1 tablespoon lemon juice or red wine vinegar
- Salt and pepper to taste
- Optional add-ins: diced bell peppers, sliced olives, crumbled feta cheese, chopped basil, or mint leaves

Instructions:

- In a large mixing bowl, combine the diced cucumbers, diced tomatoes, thinly sliced red onion, and chopped fresh parsley or cilantro.

- In a small bowl, whisk together the extra virgin olive oil and lemon juice or red wine vinegar to make the dressing.

- Pour the dressing over the cucumber and tomato mixture in the large bowl.

- Season the salad with salt and pepper to taste, and toss everything together until well combined.

- Taste the salad and adjust the seasoning if needed, adding more salt, pepper, or lemon juice/vinegar as desired.

- If using any optional add-ins such as diced bell peppers, sliced olives, crumbled feta cheese, chopped basil, or mint leaves, add them to the salad and toss to combine.

- Serve the cucumber and tomato salad immediately, or cover and refrigerate it for at least 30 minutes to allow the flavors to meld before serving.

This cucumber and tomato salad is light, refreshing, and bursting with flavor from the fresh vegetables and herbs. It's a great source of vitamins, minerals, and antioxidants, making it a nutritious option for individuals with ADHD and autism. Plus, it's versatile and easy to customize with your favorite add-ins to suit your taste preferences. Enjoy this delicious and wholesome salad as a side dish or a light meal any time of the day!

96. Sugar-free applesauce

Ingredients:
- 6-8 medium-sized apples (such as Gala, Fuji, or Granny Smith), peeled, cored, and chopped
- 1/2 cup water
- 1 teaspoon ground cinnamon (optional)

Instructions:
- In a large saucepan, combine the chopped apples and water. Bring the mixture to a simmer over medium heat, then reduce the heat to low.

- Cover the saucepan and let the apples cook for about 15-20 minutes, stirring occasionally, until they are soft and tender.

- Once the apples are cooked through, remove the saucepan from the heat and let the mixture cool slightly.

- Using a potato masher or fork, mash the cooked apples until you reach your desired consistency. For smoother applesauce, you can use a blender or food processor to puree the mixture.

- If desired, stir in ground cinnamon for added flavor. Taste the sugar-free applesauce and adjust the seasoning if needed. If the applesauce is too thick, you can stir in a little more water to reach your desired consistency.

- Transfer the applesauce to airtight containers or jars for storage. Let the applesauce cool completely before refrigerating it. It will keep in the refrigerator for up to 1 week.

Tips:
- You can adjust the sweetness of the applesauce by using sweeter apples or adding a squeeze of lemon juice to enhance the natural sweetness of the apples.

- Feel free to experiment with different spices such as nutmeg, cloves, or ginger for additional flavor variations.

- This sugar-free applesauce can be enjoyed on its own as a healthy snack, or used as a topping for oatmeal, yogurt, pancakes, or as a substitute for oil in baking recipes.

This sugar-free applesauce is a nutritious and versatile option for individuals with ADHD and autism. It's free from added sugars, preservatives, and artificial flavors, making it a wholesome choice for a variety of recipes and snacks. Enjoy the natural sweetness and flavor of apples in this delicious homemade applesauce!

97. Baked zucchini chips

Ingredients:
- 2 medium zucchinis, thinly sliced (about 1/8 inch thick)
- 1-2 tablespoons olive oil
- 1/4 cup grated Parmesan cheese (optional, omit for dairy-free or vegan)
- 1/2 teaspoon garlic powder
- 1/2 teaspoon onion powder
- 1/2 teaspoon paprika
- Salt and pepper to taste

Instructions:
- Preheat your oven to 225°F (107°C). Line a baking sheet with parchment paper or a silicone baking mat for easy cleanup.

- In a large mixing bowl, toss the thinly sliced zucchini with olive oil until evenly coated.

- In a separate small bowl, combine the grated Parmesan cheese (if using), garlic powder, onion powder, paprika, salt, and pepper.

- Sprinkle the seasoning mixture over the oiled zucchini slices, tossing to coat them evenly.

- Arrange the seasoned zucchini slices in a single layer on the prepared baking sheet, making sure they are not overlapping.

- Bake the zucchini chips in the preheated oven for 1.5 to 2 hours, or until they are crispy and golden brown, flipping them halfway through baking to ensure even cooking.

- Once the zucchini chips are crispy and golden brown, remove them from the oven and let them cool on the baking sheet for a few minutes. Serve the baked zucchini chips warm as a delicious and nutritious snack.

Tips:
- Make sure to slice the zucchini thinly and evenly to ensure that they cook uniformly and become crispy.

- Feel free to adjust the seasoning according to your taste preferences. You can experiment with different spices such as cumin, chili powder, or Italian seasoning.

- For a dairy-free or vegan option, omit the Parmesan cheese or use a dairy-free alternative.

98. Sugar-free gelatin

Ingredients:
- 1 packet (about 2 1/2 teaspoons) unflavored gelatin
- 1 cup cold water
- 1 cup boiling water
- Sugar-free sweetener of your choice (such as stevia, erythritol, or monk fruit), to taste
- Flavorings or extracts (such as vanilla, almond, lemon, or fruit extracts) as desired

Instructions:
- In a bowl, sprinkle the unflavored gelatin over the cold water. Let it sit for 1-2 minutes to soften. Stir in the boiling water until the gelatin is completely dissolved.

- Add sugar-free sweetener to taste, stirring until fully dissolved. Start with a small amount and adjust to your desired level of sweetness.

- If desired, add flavorings or extracts to the gelatin mixture for added flavor. Stir until well combined.

- Pour the gelatin mixture into molds or a shallow dish. Refrigerate the gelatin until set, which typically takes about 2-4 hours.

- Once set, remove the gelatin from the refrigerator and unmold if necessary. Serve the sugar-free gelatin cold as a refreshing and low-calorie treat.

Tips:
- Experiment with different flavors and combinations of extracts to create your favorite sugar-free gelatin flavors.

- For added texture and nutrition, you can mix in chopped fruits, berries, or nuts before refrigerating the gelatin to set.

- Adjust the sweetness level to suit your taste preferences by adding more or less sugar-free sweetener.

- To make layered gelatin, allow each layer to set in the refrigerator before adding the next layer. Store any leftover gelatin in the refrigerator for up to a few days.

This homemade sugar-free gelatin is a delicious and guilt-free dessert option for individuals with ADHD and autism, providing a satisfyingly sweet treat without added sugars or artificial ingredients. Enjoy this customizable gelatin recipe as a refreshing snack or dessert any time of the day!

99. Steamed edamame

Ingredients: Fresh edamame pods (frozen edamame can also be used)

Instructions:
- Rinse the edamame pods under cold water to remove any dirt or debris.

- If using frozen edamame, thaw them according to the package instructions.

- Bring a pot of water to a boil over high heat. Add a generous pinch of salt to the boiling water.

- Once the water is boiling, add the edamame pods to the pot.

- Cook the edamame pods for about 3-5 minutes, or until they are bright green and tender.

- Using a slotted spoon or strainer, remove the cooked edamame pods from the pot and drain them well.

- Transfer the steamed edamame pods to a serving bowl or plate.

- Sprinkle the steamed edamame pods with additional salt or seasoning if desired.

- Serve the steamed edamame pods hot or at room temperature, allowing individuals to shell and enjoy them as a nutritious snack.

Tips:
- You can customize the flavor of steamed edamame by sprinkling them with seasoning blends such as garlic powder, onion powder, chili flakes, or sesame seeds.

- To eat edamame, individuals can simply squeeze the pods to release the beans into their mouths. The pods are not typically eaten.

- Edamame can also be served cold as a chilled snack or added to salads for extra protein and texture.

Steamed edamame is rich in protein, fiber, vitamins, and minerals, making it a nutritious snack option for individuals with ADHD and autism. It's easy to prepare, versatile, and can be enjoyed as a tasty and satisfying snack any time of the day. Plus, it's fun to eat and provides a sensory experience with its unique texture and flavor. Enjoy steamed edamame as a wholesome snack or appetizer!

100. Avocado and tomato slices

Ingredients:
- 1 ripe avocado
- 1 large tomato
- Salt and pepper to taste
- Optional: Balsamic vinegar, olive oil, lemon juice, or your favorite seasoning blend

Instructions:
- Slice the avocado in half lengthwise and remove the pit. Use a spoon to scoop out the flesh from the skin.

- Cut the avocado halves into thin slices.

- Slice the tomato into thin rounds.

- Arrange the avocado and tomato slices on a serving platter or plate, alternating them or layering them if desired.

- Sprinkle the avocado and tomato slices with salt and pepper to taste.

- If desired, drizzle the avocado and tomato slices with balsamic vinegar, olive oil, lemon juice, or your favorite seasoning blend for added flavor.

- Serve the avocado and tomato slices immediately as a nutritious and delicious snack or side dish.

Tips:

- Choose ripe but firm avocados and tomatoes for the best flavor and texture.

- Feel free to customize the dish with additional toppings or garnishes such as crumbled feta cheese, chopped fresh herbs, red onion slices, or a sprinkle of chili flakes.

- Serve the avocado and tomato slices alongside grilled chicken, fish, or tofu for a balanced meal.

Avocado and tomato slices are rich in healthy fats, vitamins, and antioxidants, making them a nutritious and satisfying option for individuals with ADHD and autism. This simple dish is quick and easy to prepare, and it provides a delicious combination of flavors and textures. Enjoy avocado and tomato slices as a wholesome snack, appetizer, or side dish any time of the day!

101. Microwave scrambled eggs

Ingredients:

- 2 eggs
- 2 tablespoons milk or water
- Salt and pepper to taste
- Optional add-ins: Shredded cheese, diced vegetables, cooked bacon or sausage, chopped herbs, etc.

Instructions:

- Crack the eggs into a microwave-safe bowl. Add the milk or water to the bowl. Season the eggs with salt and pepper to taste. Use a fork or whisk to beat the eggs until well combined.

- If using any optional add-ins such as shredded cheese, diced vegetables, cooked bacon or sausage, or chopped herbs, stir them into the egg mixture.

- Place the bowl of eggs in the microwave and cook on high power for 30 seconds. Remove the bowl from the microwave and stir the eggs with a fork. Return the bowl to the microwave and cook for another 30 seconds.

- Continue microwaving and stirring the eggs in 30-second intervals until they are cooked to your desired level of doneness. The total cooking time will depend on the wattage of your microwave and how you like your eggs cooked, but it typically takes about 1-2 minutes in total.

- Once the eggs are cooked to your liking, remove the bowl from the microwave and serve the scrambled eggs hot.

Tips:

- Be careful not to overcook the eggs in the microwave, as they can become rubbery. It's better to slightly undercook them and allow them to finish cooking with residual heat.

- Feel free to customize the scrambled eggs with your favorite add-ins and seasonings to suit your taste preferences.

- Serve the microwave scrambled eggs on their own, or enjoy them with toast, a side of fruit, or your favorite breakfast accompaniments.

Microwave scrambled eggs are a convenient and protein-rich breakfast option that can be prepared in just minutes. They're perfect for busy mornings when you need a quick and nutritious meal to start your day. Enjoy these microwave scrambled eggs as a satisfying and delicious breakfast anytime!

102. Peanut butter banana sandwich

Ingredients:
- 2 slices of bread (whole wheat, multigrain, or gluten-free bread can be used)
- 2 tablespoons peanut butter (or any nut butter of your choice)
- 1 ripe banana, thinly sliced
- Optional: Honey, maple syrup, or cinnamon for added sweetness

Instructions:
- Toast the slices of bread if desired. Toasting the bread can add extra texture and flavor to the sandwich.

- Spread one tablespoon of peanut butter evenly onto each slice of bread.

- Arrange the thinly sliced banana on one slice of bread, covering it evenly with banana slices.

- If desired, drizzle honey or maple syrup over the banana slices for added sweetness, or sprinkle a pinch of cinnamon on top. Place the other slice of bread on top of the banana-covered slice to form a sandwich.

- Press down gently on the sandwich to secure the filling between the bread slices. Use a sharp knife to slice the sandwich in half diagonally or horizontally, if desired.

- Serve the peanut butter banana sandwich immediately, or wrap it in parchment paper or foil for a convenient on-the-go snack.

Tips:
- For added texture and flavor, you can sprinkle chopped nuts, shredded coconut, or chocolate chips onto the peanut butter before adding the banana slices.

- Feel free to customize the sandwich by using different nut butters (such as almond butter or cashew butter) or adding other ingredients like sliced strawberries, blueberries, or a drizzle of chocolate sauce.

- If you're making the sandwich for someone with autism who prefers certain textures, consider mashing the banana instead of slicing it for a smoother consistency.

Peanut butter banana sandwiches are a delicious and satisfying combination of flavors and textures. They're rich in protein, healthy fats, and carbohydrates, making them a nutritious and energizing snack or meal option for individuals with ADHD and autism. Enjoy this simple and tasty sandwich any time of the day!

103. Canned tuna salad

Ingredients:

- 1 can (5 oz) of tuna, drained
- 1/4 cup mayonnaise (or Greek yogurt for a lighter option)
- 1 tablespoon lemon juice
- 1/4 cup diced celery
- 1/4 cup diced red onion
- Salt and pepper to taste
- Optional add-ins: Chopped pickles, diced apples, sliced grapes, chopped nuts, or dried cranberries

Instructions:

- In a mixing bowl, combine the drained tuna, mayonnaise (or Greek yogurt), and lemon juice. Add the diced celery and diced red onion to the bowl.

- Season the tuna salad with salt and pepper to taste. If desired, add any optional add-ins such as chopped pickles, diced apples, sliced grapes, chopped nuts, or dried cranberries.

- Stir all the ingredients together until well combined. Taste the tuna salad and adjust the seasoning if needed, adding more salt, pepper, or lemon juice as desired.

- Serve the canned tuna salad immediately, or cover and refrigerate it for at least 30 minutes to allow the flavors to meld before serving.

Tips:

- Use your favorite type of canned tuna, such as chunk light tuna or solid white albacore tuna.

- You can customize the tuna salad with additional ingredients to suit your taste preferences. Experiment with different vegetables, fruits, nuts, or seasonings to create your favorite flavor combinations.

- Serve the canned tuna salad on top of lettuce leaves, whole grain bread, crackers, or as a filling for sandwiches, wraps, or stuffed tomatoes.

Canned tuna salad is a convenient and protein-rich dish that's perfect for quick and easy meals or snacks. It's packed with nutrients and flavor, making it a satisfying and nutritious option for individuals with ADHD and autism. Enjoy this versatile tuna salad recipe as a delicious and wholesome meal any time of the day!

104. Instant pot chicken and rice

Ingredients:
- 1 pound boneless, skinless chicken breasts or thighs, cut into bite-sized pieces
- 1 cup long-grain white rice, rinsed and drained
- 1 1/2 cups chicken broth
- 1 small onion, diced
- 2 cloves garlic, minced
- 1 teaspoon dried thyme
- 1 teaspoon dried oregano
- 1 teaspoon paprika
- Salt and pepper to taste
- Optional: Chopped vegetables such as carrots, bell peppers, or peas

Instructions:
- Turn on the Instant Pot and select the 'Saute' function. Heat a little oil in the pot. Add the diced onion and minced garlic to the pot. Saute for 2-3 minutes until softened and fragrant.

- Add the bite-sized chicken pieces to the pot. Season with dried thyme, dried oregano, paprika, salt, and pepper. Cook for 3-4 minutes until the chicken is browned on all sides.

- Pour in the chicken broth and deglaze the bottom of the pot, scraping up any browned bits with a wooden spoon.

- Add the rinsed and drained rice to the pot, spreading it evenly over the chicken and broth. If using any optional vegetables, add them to the pot at this point.

- Close the Instant Pot lid and set the valve to the 'Sealing' position. Cancel the 'Saute' function. Select the 'Manual' or 'Pressure Cook' setting and set the timer for 8 minutes at high pressure.

- Once the cooking time is complete, allow the Instant Pot to naturally release pressure for 10 minutes, then carefully quick-release any remaining pressure.

- Open the Instant Pot lid and fluff the chicken and rice with a fork. Check for seasoning and adjust if needed. Serve the Instant Pot chicken and rice hot, garnished with chopped fresh herbs if desired.

Instant Pot chicken and rice is a comforting and satisfying meal that's easy to prepare and packed with flavor. It's a great option for busy days when you need a quick and nutritious meal for yourself or your family. Enjoy this hearty and delicious dish as a convenient meal any time of the day!

105. No-bake energy bites

Ingredients:
- 1 cup rolled oats
- 1/2 cup nut butter (such as peanut butter, almond butter, or sunflower seed butter)
- 1/4 cup honey or maple syrup
1/4 cup ground flaxseed or chia seeds
- 1/2 cup shredded coconut (unsweetened)
- 1 teaspoon vanilla extract
- Optional add-ins: Mini chocolate chips, chopped nuts, dried fruit, cocoa powder, protein powder, or spices like cinnamon or nutmeg

Instructions:
- In a large mixing bowl, combine the rolled oats, nut butter, honey or maple syrup, ground flaxseed or chia seeds, shredded coconut, and vanilla extract.

- Stir the ingredients together until well combined. If the mixture seems too dry, you can add a little more nut butter or honey/maple syrup to help bind everything together.

- If using any optional add-ins such as mini chocolate chips, chopped nuts, dried fruit, cocoa powder, protein powder, or spices, add them to the mixture and stir until evenly distributed.

- Once the ingredients are well mixed, use a tablespoon or cookie scoop to portion out the mixture and roll it into small balls between your palms.

- Place the rolled energy bites on a baking sheet lined with parchment paper or wax paper. Chill the energy bites in the refrigerator for at least 30 minutes to firm up.

- Once chilled, transfer the energy bites to an airtight container for storage in the refrigerator. Enjoy the no-bake energy bites as a quick and nutritious snack anytime you need a boost of energy!

Tips:
Feel free to customize the energy bites with your favorite add-ins to suit your taste preferences.
Store the energy bites in the refrigerator for up to 1-2 weeks, or freeze them for longer storage.
These energy bites are portable and convenient, making them a great snack option for on-the-go or as a pre-workout or post-workout snack.

No-bake energy bites are a wholesome and satisfying snack that's packed with fiber, protein, healthy fats, and energy-boosting nutrients. They're perfect for individuals with ADHD and autism who need a nutritious and convenient snack to fuel their day. Enjoy these delicious energy bites as a tasty and satisfying treat anytime you need a quick pick-me-up!

106. Simple fruit smoothie

Ingredients:
- 1 ripe banana, peeled and sliced
- 1 cup frozen mixed berries (such as strawberries, blueberries, raspberries, or blackberries)
- 1/2 cup plain Greek yogurt (or dairy-free alternative)
- 1/2 cup milk (or dairy-free alternative)
- Optional: Honey, maple syrup, or a pitted date for added sweetness

Instructions:
- Place the sliced banana, frozen mixed berries, plain Greek yogurt, and milk in a blender.

- If desired, add a sweetener such as honey, maple syrup, or a pitted date to the blender for added sweetness.

- Blend the ingredients on high speed until smooth and creamy. If the smoothie is too thick, you can add more milk to reach your desired consistency.

- Taste the smoothie and adjust the sweetness if needed by adding more sweetener, if desired. Once the smoothie is blended to your liking, pour it into glasses and serve immediately.

Tips:
- Feel free to customize the smoothie with your favorite fruits, such as mango, pineapple, kiwi, peaches, or spinach.

- Add a scoop of protein powder, nut butter, or chia seeds for extra protein and fiber.

- For a creamier texture, use frozen banana slices instead of fresh banana.

- You can use any type of milk or dairy-free alternative in the smoothie, such as almond milk, soy milk, coconut milk, or oat milk.

Simple fruit smoothies are a refreshing and nutritious snack or breakfast option that's packed with vitamins, minerals, fiber, and antioxidants. They're easy to make and can be customized with your favorite fruits and add-ins to suit your taste preferences. Enjoy this delicious and wholesome smoothie as a quick and satisfying treat any time of the day!

107. Baked chicken breasts

Ingredients:
- 2 boneless, skinless chicken breasts
- 1 tablespoon olive oil
- Salt and pepper to taste
- Optional seasonings: Garlic powder, onion powder, paprika, Italian seasoning, or lemon pepper

Instructions:
- Preheat your oven to 375°F (190°C). Lightly grease a baking dish with olive oil or cooking spray.

- Place the chicken breasts on a cutting board and pat them dry with paper towels. This helps the seasoning adhere to the chicken and promotes even cooking. Drizzle the olive oil over both sides of the chicken breasts, rubbing it in to coat evenly.

- Season the chicken breasts generously with salt and pepper, as well as any optional seasonings of your choice.

- Place the seasoned chicken breasts in the prepared baking dish, spacing them apart so they cook evenly.

- Bake the chicken breasts in the preheated oven for 20-25 minutes, or until they reach an internal temperature of 165°F (74°C) and are no longer pink in the center. Cooking time may vary depending on the thickness of the chicken breasts.

- Once cooked through, remove the chicken breasts from the oven and let them rest for a few minutes before slicing or serving. Serve the baked chicken breasts hot as a main dish or protein component for a meal.

Tips:
- For added flavor, marinate the chicken breasts in your favorite marinade for 30 minutes to overnight before baking.

- You can add sliced onions, bell peppers, or cherry tomatoes to the baking dish for a complete meal.

Baked chicken breasts are a lean and protein-rich option that's easy to prepare and can be enjoyed in various dishes. They're a nutritious choice for individuals with ADHD and autism, providing essential nutrients for energy and focus. Enjoy these simple and delicious baked chicken breasts as part of a balanced meal any time of the day!

108. Steamed broccoli with olive oil

Ingredients:
- 1 head of broccoli, washed and trimmed into florets
- 1 tablespoon olive oil
- Salt and pepper to taste
- Optional: Lemon zest, minced garlic, grated Parmesan cheese, or red pepper flakes for added flavor

Instructions:
- Fill a large pot with a few inches of water and place a steamer basket inside. Bring the water to a boil over high heat.

- Once the water is boiling, add the broccoli florets to the steamer basket. Cover the pot with a lid and steam the broccoli for 3-5 minutes, or until it is bright green and tender-crisp. Be careful not to overcook the broccoli, as it can become mushy.

- While the broccoli is steaming, prepare the olive oil dressing. In a small bowl, whisk together the olive oil, salt, pepper, and any optional ingredients such as lemon zest, minced garlic, grated Parmesan cheese, or red pepper flakes.

- Once the broccoli is cooked to your liking, remove the steamer basket from the pot and transfer the broccoli to a serving dish. Drizzle the olive oil dressing over the steamed broccoli, tossing gently to coat evenly.

- Taste the broccoli and adjust the seasoning if needed, adding more salt, pepper, or other seasonings to taste. Serve the steamed broccoli with olive oil hot as a nutritious and delicious side dish.

Tips:
- You can customize the flavor of the olive oil dressing by experimenting with different herbs and spices, such as chopped fresh parsley, basil, or thyme.

- Feel free to add a squeeze of lemon juice over the steamed broccoli for a bright and citrusy flavor.

- Leftover steamed broccoli can be stored in an airtight container in the refrigerator for up to 3-4 days. Enjoy it cold as a salad topping or reheated as a side dish.

Steamed broccoli with olive oil is a simple yet tasty way to enjoy this nutritious vegetable. It's rich in vitamins, minerals, and antioxidants, making it a wholesome choice for individuals with ADHD and autism. Plus, it's quick and easy to prepare, making it a convenient addition to any meal. Enjoy this flavorful and nutritious side dish as part of a balanced diet!

109. Cheese and vegetable quesadilla

Ingredients:
- 4 medium flour tortillas (or gluten-free tortillas if needed)
- 1 cup shredded cheese (such as cheddar, Monterey Jack, or a Mexican cheese blend)
- 1/2 cup diced bell peppers (any color)
- 1/2 cup diced onions
- 1/2 cup sliced mushrooms
- Optional add-ins: Cooked chicken or beef strips, black beans, corn kernels, spinach, or avocado slices

Instructions:
- Heat a large skillet or griddle over medium heat. Place one flour tortilla in the skillet and sprinkle half of the shredded cheese evenly over the tortilla.

- Scatter half of the diced bell peppers, onions, and mushrooms over the cheese layer. If using any optional add-ins such as cooked chicken or beef strips, black beans, corn kernels, spinach, or avocado slices, add them on top of the vegetable layer.

- Sprinkle the remaining half of the shredded cheese over the vegetable and optional add-in layer. Place another flour tortilla on top to cover the filling, pressing down gently to adhere.

- Cook the quesadilla for 2-3 minutes on each side, or until the tortillas are golden brown and the cheese is melted and gooey. Once cooked, remove the quesadilla from the skillet and transfer it to a cutting board.

- Use a sharp knife or pizza cutter to slice the quesadilla into wedges or squares. Serve the cheese and vegetable quesadilla hot, with your favorite toppings or dipping sauces if desired.

Tips:
- You can customize the quesadilla with your favorite vegetables, cheeses, and protein options to suit your taste preferences.

- Serve the quesadilla with salsa, guacamole, sour cream, or Greek yogurt for dipping, or drizzle with hot sauce for extra flavor.

Cheese and vegetable quesadillas are a delicious and satisfying meal option that's easy to customize with your favorite ingredients. They're a great way to incorporate vegetables and protein into your diet while enjoying a flavorful and comforting dish. Enjoy these cheesy and veggie-packed quesadillas as a quick and tasty meal any time of the day!

110. Microwave sweet potato

Ingredients: 1 medium sweet potato

Instructions:
- Scrub the sweet potato under cold water to remove any dirt or debris. Pat it dry with a paper towel.

- Use a fork to prick several holes all over the sweet potato. This allows steam to escape during cooking and prevents the potato from bursting. Place the sweet potato on a microwave-safe plate.

- Microwave the sweet potato on high power for 5-7 minutes, depending on the size and thickness of the potato. If you're cooking multiple sweet potatoes at once, you may need to increase the cooking time accordingly.

- After the initial cooking time, carefully flip the sweet potato over and continue microwaving for an additional 5-7 minutes, or until the potato is tender and easily pierced with a fork.

- Once cooked, remove the sweet potato from the microwave and let it cool for a few minutes before handling. Slice the sweet potato open lengthwise and fluff the flesh with a fork.

- Serve the microwave sweet potato hot, plain, or with your favorite toppings such as butter, cinnamon, brown sugar, marshmallows, or Greek yogurt.

Tips:
- Sweet potatoes vary in size and thickness, so adjust the cooking time accordingly. A larger or thicker sweet potato may require a longer cooking time.

- Be careful when handling the sweet potato after microwaving, as it will be hot. Use oven mitts or a kitchen towel to protect your hands.

- You can store leftover cooked sweet potatoes in the refrigerator for up to 3-5 days. Reheat them in the microwave or oven before serving.

Microwaved sweet potatoes are a nutritious and versatile ingredient that can be enjoyed in various ways. They're rich in vitamins, minerals, and fiber, making them a wholesome choice for individuals with ADHD and autism. Enjoy microwaved sweet potatoes as a quick and satisfying side dish or meal any time of the day!

In "The ADHD & Autism Cookbook: 100+ Nutritious Recipes for Focus and Wellness," the author presents a comprehensive guide aimed at improving the dietary habits of individuals with ADHD and autism. The book emphasizes the crucial role nutrition plays in managing symptoms and enhancing overall well-being.

Throughout the book, readers are provided with a variety of recipes tailored to meet specific dietary needs, focusing on eliminating common allergens and incorporating nutrient-dense ingredients. These recipes are designed to support brain health, improve focus, and promote a balanced mood.

Key takeaways include the importance of:

1. Eliminating Processed Foods: Removing additives, preservatives, and artificial ingredients that may exacerbate symptoms.

2. Incorporating Whole Foods: Prioritizing fresh, organic fruits, vegetables, lean proteins, and healthy fats to provide essential nutrients.

3. Understanding Food Sensitivities: Identifying and avoiding common allergens such as gluten and dairy that may trigger adverse reactions.

4. Meal Planning: Creating structured meal plans to ensure consistency in nutrient intake and avoid potential food-related disruptions.

The book not only offers practical culinary solutions but also provides educational insights into how specific nutrients affect brain function and behavior. By integrating these dietary changes, caregivers and individuals can take proactive steps towards better health and improved management of ADHD and autism symptoms.

In summary, "The ADHD & Autism Cookbook" serves as a valuable resource, combining scientific knowledge with practical advice to help families navigate the complexities of dietary management. It underscores the profound impact of nutrition on cognitive and emotional health, advocating for a mindful, holistic approach to food and wellness.